Critics on Rick Mitchell:

...'a modern day Brecht'.
(Rosalind Friedman, *WMNR Fine Arts Radio*)

...'in its present stripped-down form, it's an uncut gem whose brilliance will
not be enhanced by additional polishing.... The fine script, superb acting,
and engaging themes combined to make (*Brecht in L.A.*) a must see
production'.
(Ralph Leck, *Communications from the International Brecht Society*)

'His work as a playwright is courageous, but never self-consciously so; there
is a recognition of the humor endemic to the situations Mitchell writes
about, as well as a recognition of the horror and absurdity'
(Elizabeth Hilts, *The Fairfield County Weekly*)

'With a wink and a nod to Bertolt Brecht, Rick Mitchell's provocative,
surrealistic play....*Ventriloquist Sex* offers a stinging critique of capitalism,
but the comedy is so funny that the audience never feels harangued....Rarely
is Theatre of Alienation so enjoyable'. (Sandra Ross, *LA Weekly*)

Author

Rick Mitchell, whose plays include *Ventriloquist Sex*, *Urban Renewal*, *Cruising the Caribbean: Old Pleasures in the New World*, *Potlatch*, and *The Gulf*, has written for stage, radio, and television, as well as for numerous journals, and his work has been produced throughout the US. He lives in Los Angeles and teaches playwriting, drama, and performance in the Department of English at California State University, Northridge. Mitchell's play *The Composition of Herman Meville* is available from Intellect Books.

Acknowledgements

I would like to thank California State University, Northridge for providing me with time to work on the first draft of *Brecht in L.A.* I am also grateful to all of the talented actors who participated in the play's initial workshopping—without them this would be a much different (and incomplete) work—as well as to my playwriting students, especially Joe Luis Cedillo, Brian Scott, and Sylvie Green Shapero, the participants in my senior seminar on Brecht and Artaud, my many supportive colleagues, Roberta Mock's editorial acumen, and, of course, the three people who make it possible for me to hole up for months at a time and knock out a script: Caroline, Christopher, and Emily.

FOR CAROLINE

Contents

Epic Theatre, Naturalistic Artifice, and American Acting: *Brecht in L.A.* in L.A.

The work must raise to the very highest level the art of quoting without quotation marks. Its theory is intimately linked to that of montage.
—Walter Benjamin, '*N*'

nowhere is writing about theatre more difficult than here, where all they have is theatrical naturalism.
—Bertolt Brecht, Los Angeles, 1 November 1941, *Journals*

Sixty-one years after Bertolt Brecht's observation, Los Angeles—which now has more small theatres than any city in the United States—often offers plays that venture beyond the strict confines of realism and naturalism.[1] In Hollywood, however, these forms have maintained a stranglehold on film and television production since the advent of the talking picture in the late 1920s. While many of the theatre artists who work here are quite capable of performing in non-realistic plays, producers of TV dramas and feature films remain primarily interested in realism. Thus, many theatre actors in Los Angeles prefer to utilize realistic acting techniques even, at times, when the play calls for a different approach. Working in a style that will help one to advance in 'the industry' is if anything practical because artists cannot pay the rent by working in low-budget, 99-seat theatres which compensate Equity actors about eight dollars per show (rehearsals not included) and often pay less (or nothing) to non-Equity actors, directors, and writers, although the influence of Hollywood—a formidable, globalizing force whose reach seems almost unlimited these days—is not the only reason for the predominance of the realistic acting style which, after all, began way back in the mid- to late-nineteenth century, as Ibsen's dramas, along with the realistic *mise-en-scènes* of directors such as Saxe-Meiningen, Andre Antoine, and, a bit later, Konstantin Stanislavsky, forever altered theatrical form.

---

[1]Historically, naturalism, a subset of realism, was, in theory, less structured and more 'scientific' than realism, since it supposedly represented onstage an objectively observed, unstructured 'slice of life'. However, both forms, critical responses to romanticism when they first appeared, are not radically different in practice, although Brecht sometimes used the term realism, which he considered to be fluid, to connote a form resembling his epic theatre. (See, for example, Brecht's *Journals*, p. 366.) I use both terms interchangeably to denote formal dramatic conventions that still remain dominant.

While numerous later theatre artists, good modernists that they were, created plays that rebelled against the new conventions, realism has maintained its hegemonic position within the realm of drama. Ironically, Brecht, whose 'anti-Aristotelian' work may have had greater impact *against* naturalistic form than the work of any other twentieth-century dramatist or director, resided in Los Angeles mid-century, spending a significant amount of his time, at least early on, attempting to sell stories to the film studios. Although Brecht's efforts met with little success, his failures here may have been more closely related to the form of his drama than its content. Contrasting the 'closed dramaturgy' of 'bourgeois drama', the sort of theatre against which Brecht was writing, with the 'open-ended dramaturgy' of Brecht's epic theatre, Darko Suvin—emphasizing the political implications of aesthetic form—observes that bourgeois drama rests

> on the twin axioms of *individualism*—conceiving the world from the individual as the ultimate reality—and *illusionism*—taking for granted that an artistic representation in some mystic way directly reproduces or 'gives' Man [and Woman] and the world. Against this Brecht took up a position of productive *critique*, showing the world as changeable, and of what I shall for want of a better term call *dialectics*: conceiving the world as a process and man [and woman] as emergent. (p. 116)

According to Suvin bourgeois drama is especially rampant in the United States where the overbearing weight of Hollywood realism—an immensely effective if often unwitting *form* of ideology consumed daily by tens of millions of television and movie viewers—makes it difficult to see beyond the dramatic fog of individualism and illusionism.[2] Hence, America seems like an inhospitable place for the playwright/director whose work resists and subverts conventions of realism, particularly when a production includes actors who believe that their primary job is to create a truthful and 'real' character,

---

[2]During the past few years reality-based TV shows such as *Cops*, *Survivor*, and *The Real World* have become increasingly popular in the United States. While the actors are amateurs whose lives are recorded throughout the day by numerous cameras, the shows that are broadcast feature protagonists and antagonists, cause and effect plots, climaxes, and (eventually) denouements. In other words, the producers stage and edit these reality-based shows so that the broadcasts adhere to basic tenets of realism. There are, of course, differences between TV dramas and reality-based TV shows—the latter don't utilize written scripts or trained professional actors, for example—but the basic structure of realism, along with its emphasis on illusionism and individualism, remains intact, albeit with slight variations.

although even a Brechtian production[3] mounted in Hollywood—the mecca of realistic acting—can benefit from competent theatre actors whose approach to acting might seem at odds, at first, with epic dramaturgy.

> *...i involuntarily look at each hill or lemon tree for a price tag. you look for these price tags on people too.*
> —B. Brecht, Los Angeles, 21 January 1942, *Journals*

As a so-called 'experimental' playwright I was aware of the potential contradictions I'd be facing once I set up shop in L.A., a city to which I moved in 1999 to teach playwriting and dramatic literature at a university in San Fernando Valley. Almost immediately after accepting the job I began thinking about Brecht, who—after fleeing across Europe from the Nazis—moved to the Los Angeles area in 1941 with his wife Helene Weigel, their two children, and his Danish mistress Ruth Berlau. Though I lacked a mistress I felt (or at least imagined) affinities with the radical, uncompromising German dramatist/director struggling to produce innovative work in a cold-war climate where the only things that seemed to matter were the bottom line and (oppressive) American nationalism. I quickly decided that I would write an 'epic' play about Brecht—who remained in the US until 1947—living and working within the shadows of Hollywood. I actually began writing the piece, *Brecht in L.A.*, in the spring of 2001 and I directed a workshop production of the play later that fall.

Originally, our company, Urban Ensemble, had planned on performing *Brecht in L.A.* as a bare-bones, off-book production but last minute personnel changes—which are more or less the norm in small-theatre productions in a city where one can actually earn a living by acting in front of the camera—made a regular production impossible. Although we came very close

---

[3]By 'Brechtian production' I mean the production of a play that utilizes/adapts (consciously or not) elements that could be attributed to Brecht's epic theatre, particularly its 'open-ended dramaturgy', while maintaining a focus on the political. The work of numerous contemporary playwrights, from Luis Valdez and Tony Kushner to Caryl Churchill and Naomi Wallace, could thus be considered Brechtian. The latter two dramatists are leading examples of playwrights who have added a feminist approach to the Brechtian arsenal which, in order to remain effective, must constantly shift along with the times. For further discussion of epic theatre and contemporary playwriting, see Wright's *Postmodern Brecht* and Reinelt's *After Brecht: British Epic Theater*.

to canceling the play after losing an actor to a movie gig a week before our scheduled opening—we had initially planned to run *Brecht in L.A.* for two weekends during EdgeFest, a Los Angeles festival of new plays by small-theatre companies, and then for four weekends thereafter—we decided at the last minute to present the piece as a staged reading for only a few shows during EdgeFest.

This was my first time putting on a play in Los Angeles (North Hollywood, to be precise) and I was quite impressed with the talent of many of our Equity-waiver actors, several of whom were career professionals with extensive film, television, and stage experience. Most of the actors whom we cast knew little if anything about epic theatre but many of them displayed considerable skills at developing characters and character relationships, concerns of naturalistic drama that Brecht disparaged in his theoretical writings (yet utilized to varying degrees in practice). These skills, combined with the *theatrical* (as opposed to illusionistic) leanings of several of the actors, helped to make my Brechtian play stronger, both in performance and within the text, which I was constantly rewriting during our five-week rehearsal period.

The rehearsal process was not without glitches, though. As often happens when I direct a new work of mine, aspects of the play were being played out in real life during the rehearsals. At times actors' personal problems mirroring their characters' problems can add an interesting level of realism to a production by blurring the lines between character and actor.[4] During *Brecht in L.A.* rehearsals, however, the primary conflicts affecting some of the actors (to whom I'll return in a moment) were not so much mirroring their characters' conflicts as undermining the non-naturalistic elements of the play and thus the play itself.

> *the infallible sign that something is not art, or that*
> *somebody does not understand art, is boredom.*
> —B. Brecht, Berlin, 28 December 1952, *Journals*

Since *Brecht in L.A.* focuses on Brecht, as well as on his relationships and ideas, it seemed appropriate to utilize a dramatic form influenced by Brecht's

---

[4]See, for example, my article 'Creating Theatre on Society's Margins' which examines the development process and performance of *Reason of Insanity*, a play I created with people with chronic mental illness who reproduced roles onstage similar to the roles that they enacted or encountered in everyday life.

epic structure, although the play's content intentionally critiques Brechtian dramaturgy at times. For example, when *Brecht in L.A.'s* title character fervently insists to Charles Laughton that theatre must eschew emotion, Brecht's heated debating seems to undermine his argument for emotional detachment. Similarly, Brecht—both in real life and in the play—believes that empathy must be banished from the stage, yet the play's Brecht is often empathetic, just as the Galileo character had been in productions overseen by the dramatist himself in spite of Brecht's insistence that Galileo never be shown in a positive light.[5] Although portrayals of Galileo that included positive, sympathetic elements clashed with his direction and theory, Brecht—who relied on intense collaboration, both onstage and off, to shape his texts—often yielded to the instincts of intelligent actors when their acting choices worked effectively onstage without undermining the production's epic *mise-en-scène*.

Nonetheless, Brecht would not allow a character to remain empathetic throughout an entire evening. Epic theatre requires that the spectator's empathy be disrupted, or 'distanced', at times because viewing a play empathetically creates an emotional bond between spectator and protagonist. Such emotional attachment, Brecht argues, precludes the critical distance which enables the spectator to think *actively* about the play's political and historical implications. A play that excludes empathy at all times, however (and it's not clear that any of Brecht's major plays excluded empathy in performance, or even within the script), may not be able to hold an audience's attention for two or three hours, which may be why Brecht, always concerned with his plays succeeding as theatre, eventually relented to his actors' insistence that Galileo be portrayed empathetically at times.

My production experience with *Brecht in L.A.* suggested that a certain degree of empathy is necessary in epic theatre. The actor who initially performed the title role during rehearsals was unwilling to portray Brecht empathetically because he believed that Brecht—both in the play and in real life—was an 'asshole'. Playing every scene with this attitude, while, ironically, an inadvertently Brechtian approach to the role since it enabled the actor to

---

[5]While Brecht often instructed his actors to eschew empathy, Laughton and Ernst Busch, both of whom played the title role in different productions of *Galileo*, did not adhere to Brecht's direction to show only the negative aspects of Galileo. As Fuegi observes, 'For Laughton in America, and for Ernst Busch in Berlin, the intensely dramatic wars between the positive and negative aspects in *Galileo* were something they insisted on keeping whatever Brecht's view as playwright/director might be' (*Chaos*, p. 91).

maintain a critical attitude towards his character, caused the actor to create a one-dimensional character who was both unlikable and uninteresting. Another actor who spent a few days with us portrayed Brecht as being completely disengaged with the world and those around him, which was even worse.

Eventually, we found a powerful actor, Brent Blair—admittedly a 'big fan' of Brecht, as well as a teacher/practitioner of Augusto Boal's very Brechtian Theatre of the Oppressed—who was able to create a character that cared about ideas, the world, relationships, although the actor, like the play itself, also showed negative sides of Brecht, and thus the sort of contradictions which are so central to Brechtian theatrical *practice*. While there are certainly reasons to dislike the Brecht of *Brecht in L.A.*, we found that if Brecht were portrayed simply as a jerk, or as someone who didn't care about anything, the audience wouldn't care about him nor, subsequently, about the play.

Although never enamored of dramatic empathy, Brecht believed that aesthetic theory should remain fluid, especially in the theatre, a highly performative space that is always in flux, changing not only from production to production of the same play, but also from night to night, moment to moment. Yet Brecht's written theory, forever frozen on the page, provides the primary path through which many scholars and artists approach the dramatist/director's work. While referring back to Brecht's theoretical statements is important, it is also necessary to examine Brecht's practice, which eschewed theoretical rigidity while utilizing various aesthetic approaches, including elements of realism, creating what John Fuegi calls a 'mixed mimetic style' (*Chaos*, p. 37):

> though he avoided use of detailed mimesis [or 'illusionism'] as a guiding principle for the whole production, he nevertheless always maintained a substantial portion of 'literal presentation' in each production[....]he would simultaneously draw attention to the theatricality of a production while providing a substantial portion of 'realistic detail'. (*Chaos*, p. 36)

Brecht's epic theatre—which he later called dialectical theatre—utilized the individualist and illusionist elements of conventional drama dialectically, showing, for example, not only the individual, but also the dialectical relationship between the individual and society, as well as other dialectical relationships, such as those between illusion and the process which makes illusion possible.

Blair, exploiting the play's mixed mimetic style, utilized empathy, but he also discarded it at times. When he abruptly broke character at the end of a scene, for example, or when he emphasized—through a critical attitude—the

6

political implications of the play and the character's actions, Blair disrupted the emotional attachment that the spectator had felt for Brecht, thereby encouraging audience members to expand their spectatorial fields of vision beyond the individualism and illusionism of bourgeois drama.

Today, of course, mixed mimetic styles can be found in numerous popular dramas (although these plays often lack the oppositional political element so crucial to Brechtian dramaturgy). One need only look at such recent American fare as *Wit* and *Side Man* to find dramatic forms that mix realistic dialogue and structure with presentational storytelling that intermittently interrupts the dialogue while breaking the fourth wall. Since the opening up of the realistic conventions of theatre is no longer unusual, American theatre actors are often capable of stepping into a Brechtian production without great difficulty. During early rehearsals of *Brecht in L.A.*, however, aspects of the play that veered from the central tenets of bourgeois drama, individualism and illusionism, proved troublesome for two experienced Hollywood actors.

One of the actors, whom I'll call D., had played numerous lead roles in films and on television and she gave a powerful cold reading of an emotionally charged scene at the audition. I offered her the part on the spot but she didn't comprehend what I had said at first, so I told her, again, that I would like her to play the role. Still seemingly unable to understand me, she said, 'Wait, I need some time to calm down before I can talk to you', and then she walked away, seemingly out of breath and in a dither. D. had become so emotionally worked up during the scene that she needed a few minutes before she would be able to communicate again.

Once we began meeting regularly, D., reluctant to utilize emotion during the daily grind of rehearsals and unwilling to approach her role in a manner that wasn't dependent on emotion, was ineffective. I was puzzled at first by the stark difference between D.'s dynamic audition and her spiritless rehearsal work, especially since her resume included impressive film credits. I came to realize, however, that while D.'s emotion-reliant approach to acting proved inefficient on the stage, it could be effective on a film set, where the performer usually acts for only a few moments at a time. Extensive psychological exploration of character can cause the actor to withdraw into the self, an insurmountable obstacle in a play which requires the characters to relate and respond to one another while telling the play's story, but a movie director has the ability to create the appearance of actors responding to each other through creative camera work, cutting, and extra takes, and she can exploit the facial effects of psychological exploration by displaying them through the close-up.

Additionally, unlike in a play, where the dialogue's pace—unfolding in real time—helps to create most of the play's overall rhythm, the rhythm of a movie is usually created in post-production through editing. Thus, the sort of acting that arose with bourgeois drama, while sometimes problematic on today's stage, can be effective in Hollywood movies, where illusionism and individualism, abetted by the technologies of mechanical and digital reproduction, continue to reign.

> *Every day, to earn my daily bread*
> *I go to the market where lies are bought*
> *Hopefully*
> *I take up my place among the sellers.*
> —B. Brecht, 'Hollywood', *Poems*

In the theatre an actor obsessed with finding her character's inner 'truth' often slows down not only the performance (as she strives to reach various emotional states), but also the rehearsal process. During our early work on *Brecht in L.A.*, for example, we focused only on the scenes that included D. and the actor who initially played Brecht, but both actors continued to ask so many questions about their characters' psychological motivations that it was not unusual to make it only half-way through a ten-minute scene during a two-hour rehearsal. Eventually, in an attempt to explain that I did not want the actors to be overly concerned with inner motivations, I paraphrased the following discussion between a flippant Brecht and writer Abe Burrows, who had been enlisted to pen the street-singer's ballad for *Galileo's* Los Angeles opening in 1947:

> *Burrows*: Tell me Bert, how does the street singer feel about Galileo?
> *Brecht*: He feels nothing.
> *Burrows*: (hesitantly) I mean...is he praising Galileo?
> *Brecht*: No.
> *Burrows*: Is he against Galileo?
> *Brecht*: No.
> *Burrows*: What do the pamphlets that he's selling say about Galileo?
> *Brecht*: They just tell about him.
> *Burrows*: (puzzled) Are they for him or against him?
> *Brecht*: It doesn't matter.

>*Burrows*: Well, just tell me one thing, Bert. Why is the man singing a song?
>
>*Brecht*: Because I want him to. (Lyons, p. 189)

In spite of my antidotes about Brecht working in Los Angeles (with which neither actor was very impressed), both actors remained resistant to elements of the play that did not adhere to their naturalistic notions of acting. When I emphasized that the actors had to find and perform the play's brisk, overall rhythm, D. said that such a task was possible only by unlocking the inner-workings of her character. 'I have to find the character's truth', she informed me. 'That's how one finds the dialogue's rhythm'.

But the dialogue's rhythm—which is *not* found in the actor's perception of a character's psychology (imagine an Elizabethan actor playing Hamlet telling Shakespeare that he has not uncovered his dialogue's rhythm because he hasn't found the inner 'truth' of his character yet)—may be at least as important to understanding a character, as well as an entire play, as psychological exploration. In an interview with John Lahr, contemporary dramatist/director David Mamet states that 'The rhythms don't just unlock something in the character...They *are* what's happening' (qtd. in Lahr, p. 78). Vsevolod Meyerhold, who had acted under Stanislavsky's direction in plays by Chekhov, a major influence on Mamet, also underlines the importance of rhythm, which he considers central to the creation of the oft-discussed atmosphere, or mood, of Chekhov's plays: 'The secret of Chekhov's mood', Meyerhold writes, 'lies in the *rhythm* of his language' (p. 320).

Although Stanislavsky's once-revolutionary system stresses that the actor must build her character by working on the character's inner life and that a play's language and setting should seem 'real', Chekhov believes that the director and actor should avoid over-emphasizing illusionism. Meyerhold, who originated the role of Trepliov in Stanislavsky's production of *The Seagull*, tells a story of Chekhov's second visit to the production's rehearsals. According to Meyerhold, one of the Moscow Art Theatre's actors told Chekhov that 'frogs were going to croak, flies to buzz, and dogs to bark' (319) during the performances. Not at all pleased with these added effects, Chekhov attempted to demonstrate to the eager actor that the intrusion of too much reality can detract from a play's art and even destroy it. As Meyerhold recounts:

>'Why all this'? asked Chekhov in a dissatisfied voice.
>
>'It's real', answered the actor.
>
>'It's real', repeated Chekhov laughing, and after a pause said: 'The stage is art. Kramskoy has a genre painting with wonderfully

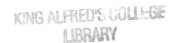

painted faces. How would it be if the nose were cut out from one of the faces and a real nose inserted? The nose will be 'real' but the painting is spoiled'. (p. 319)

Although theatre utilizes the human body as its primary medium, it still involves a great deal of artifice, *especially* in productions which attempt to reproduce a plethora of details from real life. Mamet and Chekhov, unlike Brecht, never attempt to break the fourth wall, yet all three dramatists emphasize that stage actors and directors should never confuse the artifice of the stage with the real world.

In spite of being a fan of Chekhov, D. believed that theatrical artifice had to be concealed by the 'real' at all times. Requesting 'real' props (as if props, once framed as elements in a play, are ever 'real') for rehearsals, D. announced, 'I *don't* mime'. Additionally, she kept insisting that I rewrite some of her dialogue which remained, in her view, unplayable when it wasn't 'realistic'. At certain points in the play her character—facing the audience—would deliver lines from a poem, but D. remained reluctant to address the audience directly because she could not imagine her character, at that moment in the play, speaking to a theatre audience in real life. D. also informed me that she could not walk offstage unless she knew where her character were headed:

> *D.*: 'I need to know exactly where I'm going'.
> *Director*: 'You're going backstage'.
> *D.*: 'But I need to know where my character's going'.
> *Director*: 'You're going to be out of character when you're exiting'.
> *D.*: 'Then I need a blackout'.
> *Director*: 'I didn't want to use blackouts'.
> *D.*: 'I *do not* walk across a stage when I'm out of character unless there's a blackout'.

Patiently, I tried to explain that our approach to the play was intentionally 'theatrical' and that acknowledgement of theatrical artifice was nothing new since it can be found not only in classical drama and epic theatre, but also in the work of numerous modern theatre artists. The actor continued to insist, however, that the 'truth' of the character was of utmost importance.

> *here in the states too stanislavskyism represents a protest*
> *against the commercial theatre, a handful of serious actors are*
> *building a temple, but, as it happens, on the market place.*
> —B. Brecht, Los Angeles, 15 September 1947, *Journals*

In a critique of the sort of character-centered, illusionistic acting that still remains predominant throughout much of the western world, Brecht contrasts the stylized, presentational acting of the Chinese performer with naturalistic acting that attempts to efface the fact that the person playing the onstage character is also an actor. Such effacement remains futile because no matter how earnestly a performer attempts to create the illusion of real life, the inherent duality of the actor, who is always both actor and character, can never be erased. Hence, as Brecht observes, the naturalistic actor's 'complete conversion operation is extremely exhausting' (*Brecht on Theatre*, p. 93). D., dependent on an acting technique that stressed emotion and the creation of a 'real' character, never again hit the highs and lows that she had hit during the audition. Perhaps generating strong emotions on a consistent basis while aiming for (the impossible) 'complete conversion' into the character was simply too taxing. Rather than exhaust herself or attempt a more practical acting technique, D. spent most of her rehearsal time searching for her character's elusive 'truth'.

> *there is nothing natural in art when life itself is*
> *something artificial.*
> —B. Brecht, Los Angeles, 1 November 1943, *Journals*

One could argue, as Suvin does, that illusionism and individualism remain consistent with bourgeois dramaturgy, but as such major playwrights of realism as Chekhov and Mamet suggest, a *mise-en-scène* that over-emphasizes these tenets of bourgeois drama can be damaging even to a realistic play. Mamet, for example, believes that too much concern with reaching a particular emotional state causes a theatre actor to become isolated from the rest of the ensemble, and thus from the drama:

> nothing in the world is less interesting than an actor on the stage
> involved in his or her own emotions. The very act of striving to
> create an emotional state takes one out of the play. It is the
> ultimate self-consciousness, and though it may be self-
> consciousness in the service of an ideal, it is no less boring for that.
> (pp. 10-11)

Echoing Brecht, Mamet also observes that it is ridiculous for an actor to try to transform into a 'real' character:

> The actor does not need to 'become' the character. The phrase, in
> fact, has no meaning. There *is* no character. There are only lines

upon a page. They are lines of dialogue meant to be said by the actor. When he or she says them simply, in an attempt to achieve an object more or less like that suggested by the author, the audience sees an *illusion* of a character upon the stage. (p. 9)

Contra Brecht, Mamet wants the actor to maintain a consistent 'illusion' of real life, although both dramatists believe that the actor must never attempt to circumvent a play's irrepressible artifice.

While adherents of Stanislavky's system and that related (sub)system, the Method, a partial appropriation of Stanislavsky's ideas,[6] sometimes place Brechtian dramaturgy within the enemy camp, comments by Mamet, Chekhov, and Meyerhold imply that realistic drama is not as foreign to epic theatre as many seem to believe. Mamet's and Chekhov's full-length plays, for example, fit quite comfortably within the category of realism, yet both dramatists' emphases on artifice place some of their ideas on acting closer to the philosophy of Brecht than to that of Stanislavsky. John Harrop, contrasting the Brechtian and the Stanislavskian actor, observes that:

> The acceptance of the essentially public and artificial (i.e. created by artifice) nature of theatrical performance, puts the Brechtian actor's process at the opposite end of the spectrum from the Stanislavskian actor, seen as trying too hard to build a 'real' human being from the structure of his or her own emotional responses, with which the audience will empathize... (p. 74)

Like Brecht, Mamet and Chekhov believe that the actor must accept the 'public and artificial[...]nature of theatrical performance'. The Brechtian actor, however, sets herself apart from Mamet's or Chekhov's ideal actor by building her 'role from a social perspective' (Harrop, p. 74).

Forever altering his plays and theories, Brecht believed that 'Realism'—which he considered flexible and divergent—could be useful within a progressive theatre willing to alter (and also utilize, when feasible) the form's dominant conventions. Many of Brecht's contemporaries on the left, however, radically opposed formal innovation and insisted that artists develop radical content within the dominant realistic form of the mid- to late-nineteenth century. Brecht argued that such an outmoded form would undermine any progressive content, although a fluid realism could be both radical and relevant

---

[6]For further insight into why the Method and its focus on emotional memory is only a partial and distorted rendering of Stanislavsky's acting system, see the chapter 'The Psychology in Acting' in Harrop's *Acting*. Harrop also provides an intriguing hypothesis on why the Method took such firm hold in America.

(aesthetically and politically) if its shape could continue to shift along with society's changing material conditions.[7] As Brecht writes:

> Tying a great conception like Realism to a few names is dangerous, however famous they may be, and so is the bundling together of a few forms to make a universally-applicable creative method, even if those forms are useful in themselves. Literary forms have to be checked against reality, not against aesthetics—even realist aesthetics. There are many ways of suppressing truth, and many ways of stating it. (*Brecht on Theatre*, p. 114)

Brecht blends aspects of various dramatic forms into his mixed mimetic style, creating an open-ended, self-reflexive dramaturgy that both incorporates and subverts elements of bourgeois drama.

Like some of the most powerful vehicles of ideology, the closed, illusionistic dramaturgy of conventional realism, so commonplace that we accept it as natural, acts upon us invisibly, clandestinely reinforcing dominant ways of thinking as we chew on our fingernails, fretting over the fate of the play's hero. Hence, Brecht remains adamant about the necessity of radically redefining a realism whose very form perpetuates the ideology of the status quo. As Elin Diamond points out in 'Mimesis, Mimicry, and the "True-Real"', 'Brechtian hindsight' has enabled us to realize that *conventional* realism, more than any other form,

> mystifies the process of theatrical signification. Because it naturalizes the relation between character and actor, setting and world, realism operates in concert with ideology. And because it depends on, insists on a *stability* of reference, an objective world that is the source and guarantor of knowledge, realism surreptitiously reinforces (even if it argues with) the arrangements of the world. Realism's fetishistic attachment to the true referent and the spectator's invitation to rapturous identification with a fictional imago serve the ideological function of mystifying the means of material production, thereby concealing historical contradictions, while reaffirming or mirroring the 'truth' of the status quo. (p. 366)

Citing Derrida, Diamond suggests that conventional realism (as opposed to the open, Brechtian type) 'is mimesis at its most naive—its positivist moment' (p. 366).

---

[7]For a discussion of the debates about aesthetic form between Brecht, Lukacs, a proponent of Socialist Realism, and others, see books by Wright (pp. 69-75) and Adorno, et. al. The latter book includes some of the original essays (translated into English) from the ongoing arguments.

Show that you are showing! Among all the varied
attitudes
Which you show when showing how men play their parts
The attitude of showing must never be forgotten.
—B. Brecht, from 'Showing Has to be Shown', *Poems*

A trajectory followed by *Brecht in L.A.* is Brecht's collaboration on the English adaptation of *Galileo* with Laughton, considered a 'ham' actor by Hollywood standards due to his unabashed theatricality. Brecht actually sought out such larger-than-life performers because—in addition to being entertaining—their theatricality helped to foreground the *process* of mimesis while playfully destabilizing the somber 'stability of reference' of illusionistic drama. *Galileo* opened in Los Angeles with Laughton in the lead during the summer of 1947 and shortly thereafter, with Brecht about to realize a major goal, a Broadway production, the dramatist was called to appear in front of the House Un-American Activities Committee in Washington, D.C. While he never had the opportunity to attend *Galileo's* opening on Broadway that December—Brecht quietly left America forever on Halloween, the day after his HUAC hearing—he did see another play of his in New York, the 1935 Theatre Union production of *The Mother*.

The performances of *The Mother*, however, were an utter failure because the artists of the Theatre Union, although politically radical, were unable to understand and implement the *form* of Brecht's mixed mimetic, non-naturalistic dramaturgy. According to James Lyon, when Brecht saw the initial English translation of his play by Paul Peters,

> he exploded. In his view, Peters had transformed his play into the kind of hypnotic theater [i.e., illusionism] he abhorred. The result appeared to be something resembling a well-made 'naturalistic' play, instead of what he had written as a loosely structured 'epic' piece. (p. 7)

Brecht eventually traveled to New York in a futile, infamously hostile attempt to salvage the ill-conceived production, but 'The [final] result was a hybrid production which satisfied no one' (Lyons, p. 9). While Brecht's mixed mimetic style is able to benefit from some non-Brechtian acting elements such as empathy, actors and directors working within the Brechtian form must *also* critique and disrupt empathy, as well as individualism and illusionism. Apparently, *The Mother* was unable to withstand an interpretation that was closer to bourgeois drama than epic theatre.

Collaboration with competent, open-minded theatre artists can help to strengthen an open-ended play, but as the Theatre Union's production of *The Mother* suggests, resistance to such a play's non-naturalistic elements can produce obverse results. When I was working on the production of my own

play, the two actors who found *Brecht in L.A.'s* Brechtian aspects problematic
were never able to adapt to the play's open-ended style. I could have placated
these actors by making some of their scenes more realistic, but that would have
radically altered the play, resulting perhaps in the sort of 'hybrid' production of
The Mother that had failed so miserably in New York. It seemed more prudent
to find two new actors. Fearing that I'd be unable to secure a suitable male
actor to play Brecht (with a German accent) on short notice, I opted to replace
only D., the actor most resistant to Brechtian dramaturgy. Not unexpectedly,
the actor playing Brecht, who had developed a tight bond with D., resigned
shortly thereafter. Unsure of how the remaining cast members would respond
at our next rehearsal, I was relieved when most of the other actors gladly
welcomed the cast changes, even though we were without 'a Brecht' for the
moment. Fortunately, Blair—a specialist in dialects—became available to play
Brecht a week or so later.

Always aware of the dialectical requirements of epic theatre, Blair was the
production's most Brechtian actor. The other actors, focusing more on their
characters and not as much on the play's non-naturalistic and social aspects, did
not, however, detract from the play's Brechtian *mise-en-scène*. Their
empathetic renderings of their characters helped to deepen the complexity of
the play, and the theatricality of some of the actors drew attention to process, at
least indirectly, while the play's frequent display of written quotations (during
the staged readings we used placards rather than projections) and narrative
interruptions (accomplished, for example, through numerous short scenes and a
character who observed and commented on Brecht's behavior to Brecht), along
with Blair's dialectical portrayal of the title character, enabled the play to
maintain its open-ended form. Performing the piece as a staged reading also
helped to display the play's constructedness. One critic wrote that seeing the
actors perform the play on-book was preferable to watching a regular
production, since the actors' visible reading (many of the actors actually only
glanced at the script) enhanced the play's Brechtian form by emphasizing the
process that underlies the illusion.[8]

> *the idea that matters of concern to the nation might be treated
> on the stage is utterly fanciful, since nothing of the kind happens
> anywhere else in the entertainment business.*
> —B. Brecht, Los Angeles, 27 December 1941, *Journals*

Holed up in Zurich after fleeing America, Brecht concentrated on writing
his longest theoretical treatise, 'A Short Organum for the Theatre', while
seeking a home for his work in East Berlin. In the 'Organum' Brecht tempers
many of his theories about drama, making them a bit less confrontational and

---

[8]See Appendix II, where the review, 'Brecht, Bobos, & L.A.', has been reprinted.

somewhat more accepting of certain dramatic conventions, although Brecht
continues to emphasize the importance of open-ended form. First and
foremost, however, theatre must be pleasurable: 'From the first it has been
theatre's business to entertain people, as it also has of all the other arts. It is
this business which always gives it its particular dignity; it needs no other
passport but fun, but this it has got to have' (*Brecht on Theatre*, p. 180). Yet
'fun' is not necessarily sufficient in itself; art consists of 'weaker (simple) and
stronger (complex) pleasures' (p. 181) and Brecht prefers the latter: 'The last-
named, which are what we are dealing with in great drama, attain their
climaxes rather as cohabitation does through love: they are more intricate,
richer in communication, more contradictory and more productive of results'
(p. 181).

While Brecht's theoretical writings often oppose the dominant conventions
of bourgeois drama, there are parallels between Brechtian and naturalistic
dramaturgy. Angelika Hurwicz, who acted under Brecht's direction at the
Berliner Ensemble, makes comments about acting for Brecht in the 1950s that
could equally apply to working under Mamet's direction in the early twenty-
first century. 'Abstract psychology', she writes, 'is unimportant' (p. 133), and
despite Brecht's complex theoretical writings, Hurwicz suggests that his theatre
is actually quite simple. 'To play epic theatre means to tell the story of the
play. All the work is subordinated to this end' (Hurwicz, p. 133). Mamet's
ideal actor, whose first responsibility is 'to tell the story simply' (Mamet, p.
109), possesses skills that could be useful for performing a Brechtian character,
although in order to help produce the richly communicative, 'contradictory'
results that one finds in great epic drama the actor would also have to break the
hypnotic trance of illusionism, at least intermittently, while showing that the
world is created by people, just like the spectators in the audience, who are also
capable of transforming the world.

America lacks a strong tradition of open-ended political dramaturgy, but all
drama is inherently theatrical (and political) in spite of the individualism and
illusionism that seek to snuff out any inkling of process. Some actors,
unwilling to challenge the ideology of form, refuse to embrace drama's
inherent theatricality, although the many complementary elements that one
finds in the work of Brecht, Stanislavsky, and numerous other theatre artists
ensconced in the modern canon—such as Chekhov and Mamet—suggest that
the contemporary production of plays that embrace open-ended dramaturgy is
quite feasible here. Yet the hegemony of illusionistic realism, strengthened by
its complicity with the dominant ways of thinking, Hollywood, and an
increasingly oppressive American government, remains formidable, especially
today, which is why the development of effective, Brechtian-type
dramaturgical practices in the United States may be more important than ever
before.

Rick Mitchell

i am listening to schonberg's 'theme with 7 variations' on the radio when the doorbell rings. an anaemic, prematurely aged young woman on the doorstep asks, 'can i ask you for busfare'? i hastily give her ten cents and go on listening to the romantic work with its pre-stabilised harmony.
—B. Brecht, Los Angeles, 21 October 1944, _Journals_

Brecht in L.A.

Characters (in order of appearance)

Ruth Berlau
Angel
Bertolt Brecht
Tom
Fritz Lang
Charles Laughton
Elsa Lanchester
Marshal (male; can be played by an actor who's playing another role)

(If some actors play more than one role—i.e., if the actor playing LAUGHTON also plays LANG, the actor playing TOM also plays the MARSHAL, and if the actor playing BERLAU also plays LANCHESTER—the play can be performed with five actors.)

Setting

Los Angeles County. 1940s.
(Brief scenes in Copenhagen, New York, and Washington, D.C.)

Note: *Brecht in L.A.* must be played at a brisk pace, and the set should be somewhat abstract so that there's little or no down time between scenes. Additionally, productions may utilize video imagery to subvert and/or enhance the on-stage action. (If you use video, avoid—as much as possible—imagery that has too literal of a connection to the stage action.) Also, several of the characters, especially the men, are often smoking—or at least handling—cigars. (The size of a character's cigar may increase or decrease as his/her power increases or decreases.) As far as the character of BRECHT goes, it is important that BRECHT seems vulnerable at times, that he cares about many of the people around him, about the world, ideas. In spite of Brecht's many essays that call for a theatre without emotion, the character BRECHT should often be empathetic. When a character's line ends with '—' the following character should speak over the previous character's last words. And there are numerous other times throughout the text where slight overlapping of dialogue (and/or a compression of time/space between lines) will help the actors to play the proper 'rhythm' of the piece (which is crucial). When working on this play, please keep in mind Brecht's advice to the players of the Berliner Ensemble: 'Keep it quick, light and strong'.

Brecht in L.A. was first performed on 11 November 2001 as a staged reading, directed by Rick Mitchell, as part of the Edge of the World Theater Festival, Los Angeles, at the Bitter Truth Playhouse, with the following cast:

RUTH BERLAU	Mary Beth O'Donovan
ANGEL	Del Toro
BERTOLT BRECHT	Brent Blair
TOM	Brian Scott
FRITZ LANG	Jon Peterson
CHARLES LAUGHTON	Edmund Shaff
ELSA LANCHESTER	Catherine McGoohan
MARSHAL	Jon Peterson

ACT I

PROLOGUE

(Throughout much of the play, ANGEL may sit in a far corner of the stage, at a workbench full of books and manuscripts, rolling cigars. LIGHTS UP on BERLAU, who unfolds a poem written on a well-worn piece of paper.)

BERLAU   From a poem by Bertolt Brecht...to me, Ruth Berlau...

I've longed for love engulfed by fire,

Yet resistant to becoming ash.

We both complete the other's desires,

As we're burning, but never yearning,

For ash. *(As BRECHT holds a bag of groceries he embraces BERLAU; they are looking up at the stars.)*

ANGEL   A winter evening, Copenhagen.

BRECHT   *(BRECHT points to some stars.)* Do you see it now?

BERLAU   What?

BRECHT   The letter?

ANGEL   Mid 1930s.

BERLAU   *(pause)* No.

BRECHT   Right there... The W.

BERLAU   Oh, okay... I think I see it.

BRECHT   Right up there. *(BRECHT draws a slanted W in the air.)*

BERLAU   Yes, yes...

BRECHT   Cassiopeia has five stars. And that's ours, in the middle. Where both sides come together... From now on, whenever we're apart, we'll always meet up there.

BERLAU   Up in heaven...

BRECHT   All right? *(BERLAU laughs, kisses BRECHT.)*

BERLAU   But heaven's not real.

BRECHT   The star's real. You can see it.

BERLAU   It's unattainable.

BRECHT   But it's always there. Burning.

BERLAU   I need something I can hold.

BRECHT   Here, you can carry the groceries. *(BRECHT hands her the grocery bag.)*

BERLAU   Too bad you can't carry me. *(BRECHT scoops her up.)* Aaahhh... Brecht, be careful. There are eggs in there.

SCENE ONE

(BRECHT'S front yard.)

(Discretely, under partial cover, TOM—the BRECHTS' next-door neighbor—may periodically scan the scene in front of BRECHT'S house with a telescope, other surveillance devices, throughout much of the play. BRECHT, with an open loaf of Wonderbread on his lap, is eating a slice of bread. A pile of mail sits next to him. BERLAU works, rakes, takes notes. BRECHT smokes a cigar. Note: scene settings may be projected or announced by ANGEL.)

ANGEL   Los Angeles, California. 1940s.

BRECHT   Proper bread cannot be sliced and then sit in a waxed-paper wrapper for several weeks.

BERLAU   It's the only one you haven't tasted yet.

BRECHT   All I want is proper German bread... I'd even take French...Italian...

BERLAU   Brecht, you've already tried that.

BRECHT   No, I've tried *American* versions of French and Italian. Which, underneath the bright fluorescent lighting, look decent enough. So you pick it up while it's still warm, plop it on the dinner table... Slice off the end... And then the inside, it just crumbles. Or the knife doesn't cut through at first. It just pushes down on the crust, like you're cutting into a sponge. There's nothing beneath the surface but *scheisse*. *(BERLAU intermittently rakes.)* And people work too hard around here to cover up the desert...

BERLAU   The garden looks like shit.

BRECHT   How am I supposed to get any writing done if I have to water the grass twice a day... Make sure everything looks neat, perfect. Better than real life, but lifeless... Like a goddamn corpse at a wake... Like this neighborhood of hideous stucco boxes...enormous garages with living quarters built onto the back. Even these houses, they make them to last fifteen years...out of mud and chicken wire... Nothing has any permanence here. For inspiration, I like to stroll through plazas. But there aren't any. Nobody even walks. A writer needs to feel history, change. But it never gets cold. It never rains. The trees barely shed their leaves... Cease paying the water company, and the lawn turns brown. And everyone's worrying about our yard as Hitler's butchery decides the fate of Europe sixteen thousand kilometres away. While we sit here and wither. Where the weather's always cheerful. Dry, bright, happy... Everybody's always so happy. Because they're too influenced by all this sunshine...which so dehydrates the brain that the writers who move out here end up only being able to churn out mindless drivel. So maybe if I keep sitting outside I'll soon write something acceptable to Hollywood...so I can afford to maintain my goddamn grass.

BERLAU	Where are the rest of the gardening tools?
BRECHT	In the garage.
BERLAU	Here. *(BERLAU hands BRECHT some notes.)*
BRECHT	What's this?
BERLAU	Some ideas for a film about bread.
BRECHT	We have to write about workers.
BERLAU	The film examines a German breadmaker...
BRECHT	If I don't sell something quickly, I'm going to lose my fucking house. *(BRECHT pockets notes.)*
BERLAU	You have to convince Laughton to play Galileo.
BRECHT	It needs a better translation.
BERLAU	I've spent over six months on that.
BRECHT	We just need someone who's a bit more familiar with the nuances of English...
BERLAU	Well, perhaps a few of the idioms could be improved.
BRECHT	I'd like to rewrite the entire play.
BERLAU	The Swiss production was very successful. *(BERLAU continues working.)*

BRECHT   The world's changed in the past few years. *(BRECHT watches BERLAU work, eventually embraces her.)* You know, you're even more attractive when you're proletarian.

BERLAU   I'm attracted to proletarians, too.

BRECHT   Wonderful. *(BRECHT pulls her close, kisses her.)*

BERLAU   But I also like you for some reason. *(BERLAU pushes away.)*

BRECHT   Certainly, my writing advances the cause of the worker—

BERLAU   I'm going to go trim the hedges. *(BERLAU begins to leave.)*

BRECHT   You'll save me some work.

BERLAU   I'll save your wife some work. *(BRECHT writes and reads a bit. BERLAU works. BRECHT reads BERLAU'S notes, jots down some words in his notebook. TOM puts away telescope, ENTERS BRECHT'S yard, stops, watches BRECHT write, walks up to BRECHT.)*

TOM   Hey, there... *(BRECHT looks up.)* I live right next door, in the blue bungalow... *(BRECHT continues writing.) (pause)* Are you a writer? *(BRECHT nods yes.)* Hey, so am I... I just started getting really serious about it a couple of months ago... *(TOM sniffs the air.)* What's that smell?

BRECHT   I don't smell anything. *(TOM tries to discretely smell his hands, armpits. Throughout scene, he tries to discern where smell is coming from.)*

TOM   What are you working on?

BRECHT   Well, I have several projects...

TOM   *(Sticking his finger on BRECHT'S notebook.)* What's that?

BRECHT   A poem. *(BRECHT takes out and looks over a manuscript.)*

TOM   Hey, that's great. I'm working on my first book right now: 'Hope'. The main story's about this boy who's a genius. But he's also poor and can't quite get it together, until his dad takes him to this conference on patriotism in Omaha sponsored by the Baptist Church and the FBI... What are you reading?

BRECHT   *(pause)* A future book of mine.

TOM   Hey, I read books, too... *(BRECHT gives quick, disinterested smile.)* Hey...you know how sometimes when you're in a book store, just checkin' things out, how a particular book just reaches out and grabs you by the throat?

BRECHT   *(pause)* No.

TOM   Hey, what's your name, by the way?

BRECHT   Brecht.

TOM   Breath?

BRECHT   Brecht.

TOM   Nice to meet you, Breath. I'm Tom. *(TOM shakes BRECHT'S hand.)* You know what I love about L.A.? There are just so many artists here... Everywhere... I mean, I know this guy...he's been comin' to where I work, Hollywood Bowl, for about five years. Always says hello. And I just found out he was the producer of *Tarzan Finds a Son*. And he didn't even know I was a writer... He told me to get him a script... I like what...what I think Orson Welles said, 'A man's gotta walk his own straight and narrow path'... You do that and good things happen, you know. I'm even getting into performing now. You see, there was this show comin' up at the Bowl, 'Roman Holiday', and the director, he asked me if I wanted to be a Trojan. I said, 'You want me to play a condom'? He said, 'No, a Trojan soldier'. *(BERLAU ENTERS, continues yardwork.)* Hey, I don't mean to be rude or anything, but I really gotta get home so I can get some writing done. But it was great talkin' to you, and I'll make sure I stop by again sometime.

BRECHT   *Ja. Hoffentlich.*

TOM   What?

BRECHT   Yes.

TOM   Are...are you German? *(BRECHT nods yes.)* From Germany?

BRECHT   Correct.

TOM   That's not your wife...

BRECHT   A friend.

TOM	You know, if I hadn't stopped over here I would have never known that I had a neighbor straight from Germany...
BRECHT	Well, there were a few detours...
TOM	What sort of detours?
BRECHT	Denmark, Russia...
TOM	Russia?
BRECHT	Yes.
TOM	You were in Russia?
BRECHT	Just before leaving for America.
TOM	Do you wanna go back?
BRECHT	When the war's over.
TOM	I guess you can't go back any sooner.
BRECHT	Not with the Nazis in power.
TOM	Nazis aren't exactly welcome in the US.
BRECHT	I would hope not.
TOM	And neither are Communists. *(BERLAU ENTERS, working. She nears BRECHT.)*
BRECHT	There are many different forms of Nazism. *(TOM notices letter postmarked in Mexico.)*
TOM	What's that?
BRECHT	What?
TOM	*(TOM points to an item of mail.)* That envelope.
BRECHT	Why?
TOM	Oh...I was just noticing that...that unusual postmark... Pohs-stal-ee???
BERLAU	*Postale*. It's Spanish.
TOM	*(To BERLAU.)* You're Mexican?
BERLAU	Danish. I lived in Spain for a while.
BRECHT	The letter's from Mexico... *(BERLAU returns to her work.)*
TOM	*(To BRECHT.)* You must know people from everywhere.

BRECHT	*(BRECHT holds up letter.)* This is just an acquaintance from the Free German movement.
TOM	*(TOM smiles.)* Well, good meeting you, friend... *(BRECHT smiles, nods. TOM EXITS. BRECHT reads, writes, as BERLAU continues working. Eventually, ANGEL ENTERS smoking a fat cigar, surveying yard.)*
ANGEL	*(To BERLAU.)* Is this your house?
BERLAU	It's his.
ANGEL	*(To BRECHT.)* I'd like to help you with the lawn.
BRECHT	I don't need any help.
ANGEL	Everything's overgrown.
BRECHT	The lawn's fine.
BERLAU	This is the last time I'm doing yardwork. *(BERLAU EXITS, continues working.)*
BRECHT	*(To ANGEL.)* I can take care of it myself.
ANGEL	No problem. *(ANGEL begins to leave.)*
BRECHT	How much?
ANGEL	*Vamos a ver... (Purveys yard.)* I can take care of the grass, shrubs...weeds...for a very low price.
BRECHT	How much?
ANGEL	*(pause)* Ten...ten dollars a month.
BRECHT	That's too high.
ANGEL	I gotta eat.
BRECHT	I understand that... But I was recently forced to move here from another country.
ANGEL	So was I.
BRECHT	So I don't have much income right now. But if you can take care of the entire garden, and do it well...I can pay you five.
ANGEL	*(ANGEL laughs.)* Five dollars? For all this?
BRECHT	Well, you don't need to trim the shrubs and weed every time you're here...
ANGEL	It's easier I do it every week.
BRECHT	Suit yourself.

ANGEL   *Tengo gasolina, mi troca, máquinas—*

BRECHT   I'll give you seven.

ANGEL   I can start off at eight. But beginning next month, you pay ten.

BRECHT   The garden's so small...I'm sure it won't take any time at all.

ANGEL   Why you don't do it yourself?

BRECHT   I, uhhh...I would. But I have too much work.

ANGEL   You work for nothin'?

BRECHT   Well, no... I mean, I try not to... But I'm a writer.

ANGEL   You need to smoke a *puro, señor.*

BRECHT   At least the average person can afford a five-cent cigar. *(BRECHT holds up his cigar.)*

ANGEL   In Cuba, the master cigar maker rolls only the finest tobacco...freehand, without any molds or *máquinas.* The primary tools *son las manos. (BRECHT periodically jots down notes.)*

BRECHT   Without mechanization, workers can't buy cigars.

ANGEL   Machines are causing workers to lose their jobs.

BRECHT   The problem is who owns them.

ANGEL   It doesn't matter.

BRECHT   If workers owned the means of production, they wouldn't be exploited.

ANGEL   The rhythm of the machines, their noise, destroys the work place... They make it impossible to think... In Cuba, before the *fascistas* took power, before cigar machines proliferated, there were lecterns in the cigar workroom. *Y todo el día,* the workers were able to listen to readings of *la literatura,* political philosophy... The stories of workers, the *pensamientos* of Marx, Neruda, Martí read from the lectern, affected the rhythms of the work. And traces of the readings clung to the craftsmen's *puros*...the way the handprints of the sculptor cling to the clay bust. *(ANGEL checks a tool or two of his gardening trade.)*

BRECHT   This whole idea of workers learning reminds me of my epic theatre, which encourages the spectator to transform the—

ANGEL   *(ANGEL looks at watch.)* I have to go mow a lawn.

BRECHT	When can you start working for me, uh...what's your name?
ANGEL	Angel. I come every Friday. First thing in the morning.
BRECHT	And I'm paying you seven dollars a month.
ANGEL	Eight.
BRECHT	Eight?
ANGEL	You said eight.
BRECHT	Fine. Eight dollars a month.
ANGEL	And then ten.
BRECHT	Once I start making sufficient income...
ANGEL	I own my own lawnmower, *señor*, so you cannot exploit me, correct?
BRECHT	But I own the land. Although, of course, I'm going to treat you fairly—
ANGEL	*Buenas tardes, señor. (BERLAU continues trimming, BRECHT writes.)*
BERLAU	Here. *(She hands the hedge clippers to BRECHT.)*
BRECHT	What's the matter?
BERLAU	My hands are starting to blister. *(BRECHT gets amorous.)*
BRECHT	That's nothing that a good fuck can't clear up.
BERLAU	Your wife and children are in the house.
BRECHT	We'll go to your place.
BERLAU	*(BERLAU hands hedge clippers to BRECHT.)* Why don't you finish up?
BRECHT	I have get to my meeting. *(BRECHT puts on his cap.)*
BERLAU	You've been wearing the same shirt and pants for the past two days.
BRECHT	I'm stopping by later tonight to finish the play.
BERLAU	Tonight won't work.
BRECHT	Why not?
BERLAU	I have plans.
BRECHT	With who?
BERLAU	I have to go out.
BRECHT	Where?
BERLAU	To the laundromat... Maybe you can help.
BRECHT	I'll stop by tomorrow night.

BERLAU   Maybe you shouldn't stop by at all.

BRECHT   Ruth, I'm sorry I haven't been able to make it over the past few nights... But
          whenever I'm not around...you have to put on that white nightgown I gave you,
          look up at our star... Which, like me, will always be there.

BERLAU   The star hasn't come out since we moved to Los Angeles.

BRECHT   It must be the smog.... C'mon. *(EXEUNT.)*

(**Projection**: FBI file on B. Brecht: Since correspondence between the Free German group in Mexico and persons in the Los Angeles area has been carried on...it is recommended that the following subjects be placed on the National Censorship Watch List for ninety days: 1. [blacked out]. 2. [blacked out]. 3. Bertolt Brecht, 1063-26 Street, Santa Monica, California.)

SCENE TWO

(FRITZ LANG'S office.)

(LANG smokes a huge cigar, BRECHT a small one.)

LANG   In America, donuts will have a much stronger appeal than bread.

BRECHT   Donuts are going to detract from the movie's gestus.

LANG   It's what?

BRECHT   Social commentary...

LANG   You were talking about a loaf of bread.

BRECHT   If the audience can be made to see a loaf of bread in a radically different light,
          then they might see the world differently—

LANG   Just give me the story.

BRECHT   It's the Depression. The father's a wheat farmer—from Kansas, destitute, living
          in Chicago... And the family's tired of waiting in bread lines... Especially
          because the mother's bread is so much tastier than any bread from the city...

LANG   Why don't you change it to jelly donuts?

BRECHT   No.

LANG   Glazed crullers.

BRECHT   *(Adamantly.)* It's bread or nothing.

LANG   You know...I've been here too fucking long... And...I've tried. And I still try. To create something substantive. But it's like slamming my head into a fucking brick wall.

BRECHT   Lang, you've done incredible work...*M, Metropolis—*

LANG   In Germany! Here, you do the best you can while dealing with censors, the American government. Which thinks that all Jews are Communists... *(Looks at watch.)* And I have to go right now. Because they want me to direct a melodrama about a sideshow contortionist who becomes a pin-up girl... And I have to attend a meeting with the 'star', who can't remember her lines because she drinks Grand Marnier all day. But the film's going to get made. You know why? Because Americans go to the cinema to see fucking movie stars. *(LANG begins to EXIT.)*

BRECHT   Could you use my wife for an acting role?

LANG   Helly?

BRECHT   Yeah.

LANG   Her accent's too strong.

BRECHT   You're making movies about Nazis.

LANG   The only Germans we ever show are soldiers. But if the studio wants me to cast a female Nazi, I'll recommend your wife. *(LANG EXITS.)*

BRECHT   I'm sure she'll appreciate it.

(Projection:
Scratch the too-green lawn
and find the truth of the place:
arrid sand, a lizard.
Or walk along the once mighty L.A. River,
and peruse a victory over nature:
a dry canal of white cement,
well-worn mattresses, broken tires,
a stagnant trickle of sewage pesticide motor oil.

Throughout this sprawling city
there's no shortage of luxuries for all,

i.e., endless backyards,
containing swimming pools
that are constructed for joyous people
and therefore remain vacant
even when brimming with swimmers.
—bb)

SCENE THREE

(LAUGHTON'S house.)

LAUGHT.   What we need is art. Art! *(LAUGHTON spills his whiskey.)* Now you're probably thinking, this actor...he has a villa high on the hill in Pacific Palisades, overlooking the sea... Two full refrigerators, antiques, rare paintings, foreign automobiles... How can he complain? Pour me another one, will you? *(BRECHT pours drink.)* Well, I'll tell you... If I just go with the flow, continue working with Hollywood hacks...I'm whoring myself. And fifty years from now, my possessions, my work...it won't mean squat to anyone.

BRECHT   *(BRECHT coughs periodically throughout scene.)* I realize that the material you've had to deal with hasn't always been...first rate.

LAUGHT.   At the moment I'm playing a bloke from the Australian outback who adopts several orphans...

BRECHT   Sounds like a real tear-jerker.

LAUGHT.   The children, they're constantly running around, hanging on my arms and legs. But I don't know how to deal with children... To tell you the truth, I can't stand them. And the script, it's full of syrupy sentiment.

BRECHT   That's what Americans want.

LAUGHT.   It's what the studios want... I wish you could have seen my stage work.

BRECHT   Even in your films, Laughton, one can tell you're an artist of the theatre, steeped in the Elizabethan tradition.

LAUGHT.   Well, I *am* English.

BRECHT   Your acting suggests control, yet vulnerability... A critical attitude towards the material...

LAUGHT.	This Galileo of yours, I think he's right up there with Lear, Hamlet.
BRECHT	Why don't you play the lead?
LAUGHT.	Oh, I wouldn't have the slightest idea of how to begin.
BRECHT	You have to play Galileo. On Broadway. You'd be perfect.
LAUGHT.	I'm honored, Bert... May I call you Bert?
BRECHT	Well, actually most people—
LAUGHT.	But I'm afraid I have several films scheduled.
BRECHT	We'll work around them. And we need to get you a better translation.
LAUGHT.	Have you met William Faulkner yet?
BRECHT	The revision needs an actor, not a novelist. Someone who can make the English language work in performance. Which is why I think you ought to collaborate with me.
LAUGHT.	I'm not a writer.
BRECHT	Don't you rewrite your film scripts?
LAUGHT.	Well, some of my lines. But I do it on the set. In the midst of rehearsing, or between takes...
BRECHT	That's exactly how writing should be done. With actors, a stage...
LAUGHT.	I think Galileo could use a bit more passion.
BRECHT	Passion gets in the way of thinking.
LAUGHT.	Good scientists are passionate about their work.
BRECHT	There cannot be any emotion in epic theatre.
LAUGHT.	Then why would the spectator care about Galileo?
BRECHT	The spectator has to think.
LAUGHT.	Right, about the character.
BRECHT	About history, about Galileo's concerns as today's concerns.
LAUGHT.	There needs to be more tension.
BRECHT	There's tension between property owners, the poor. The Church and Galileo.
LAUGHT.	I think Galileo has a big appetite—for knowledge, food, drink. He likes physical comfort. And if you place greater emphasis on the dichotomy between science and the flesh, body and soul, then you'll—

35

BRECHT	What's soul?
LAUGHT.	Human spirit.
BRECHT	What's that?
LAUGHT.	Read the Bible.
BRECHT	'Spirit' is nothing but an abstraction.
LAUGHT.	It's what infuses Art.
BRECHT	The play is about who controls knowledge. How it's used, concealed, manipulated.
LAUGHT.	The story's about people.
BRECHT	But unless the audience can see them as agents and objects of history, we might as well be writing a script for Abbott and Costello.
LAUGHT.	The play's based on reality, right?
BRECHT	Reality has many versions.
LAUGHT.	Any truthful play is based in the real world.
BRECHT	Of course.
LAUGHT.	And you live in the real world.
BRECHT	I live in Los Angeles.
LAUGHT.	And you get emotional at times... Emotion's part of reality.
BRECHT	But a stage production is not reality. It's rehearsed, written, planned out ahead of time.
LAUGHT.	Individuals still get emotional.
BRECHT	Not in a play that's going to change the way people think.
LAUGHT.	*(pause)* Look, Bert, I'm not a theorist. I'm an artist. And I'm sure that this script could make for powerful theatre. But I can only play the role if I have some control over my character. *(BRECHT picks up a small statue.)*
BRECHT	Well, I'm certainly not averse to intelligent input.
LAUGHT.	Do you have a director yet?
BRECHT	No.
LAUGHT.	What about Orson Welles?
BRECHT	Well, uh...*Citizen Kane* wasn't bad.

36

LAUGHT.	I want you to send him a copy of *Galileo Galilei*.
BRECHT	What's this?
LAUGHT.	Oh, I collect pre-Colombian art.
BRECHT	It looks like...two men fucking.
LAUGHT.	Well, there are many different types of passions.
BRECHT	*(pause)* The lovers' faces show absolutely no emotion.
LAUGHT.	Fucking doesn't have to be passionate.
BRECHT	Exactly.
LAUGHT.	But it's much more fun when it is.
BRECHT	But when it's demonstrated, as art, it has to be controlled.
LAUGHT.	Sit down. *(LAUGHTON gestures to couch.)* Let me get you another beer.
BRECHT	*(BRECHT looks at watch.)* No.
LAUGHT.	How about some oysters on the half-shell?
BRECHT	Some other time.
LAUGHT.	At least let me get you an aperitif for the road.
BRECHT	I can't take any chances.
LAUGHT.	A shot of Sambuca's not going to impair your driving.
BRECHT	I'm an 'enemy alien', Laughton. If they catch me outside after eight o'clock, they're going to shoot me...lock me up.
LAUGHT.	*(LAUGHTON looks at his watch.)* It's not going to take you an hour to get home.
BRECHT	I don't trust the traffic.
LAUGHT.	You'll be fine.
BRECHT	And I, uh...I promised the children I'd listen to the boxing match with them on the radio. *(BRECHT gets up, puts on cap.)*
LAUGHT.	Well, I really wish you could stay a bit longer... But I'm glad you stopped over. *(LAUGHTON hugs BRECHT and shakes his hand.)*
BRECHT	What are you doing tomorrow?
LAUGHT.	I have to be on the set.
BRECHT	Why don't you come by the house when you're done?

LAUGHT.   Oh, I'll be exhausted.

BRECHT   How about Saturday?

LAUGHT.   *(LAUGHTON checks his date book.)* I can't make it till after dinner.

BRECHT   I'll put on a pot of coffee.

LAUGHT.   Fine. As long as they don't call us into Warner Brothers.

BRECHT   Didn't they just go on strike this morning?

LAUGHT.   *(pause)* One of the technicians' unions.

BRECHT   You didn't cross a picket line...

LAUGHT.   Well, I...I didn't want to. And I held out... As long as I possibly could... I stayed outside the gate talking with the workers for almost an hour... And I was just about to turn around and go home when this new assistant producer showed up... Actually, he seemed more like a gangster.

BRECHT   He probably was.

LAUGHT.   He told me that anyone who honored the picket line was considered a Communist sympathizer. *(BRECHT laughs.)*

BRECHT   The studios are bringing in the mafia to break the unions now, contain the spread of socialism... All while ensuring the impossibility of democracy. *(BRECHT laughs.)*

LAUGHT.   Then you appreciate the difficulty of my position?

BRECHT   No, I don't.

LAUGHT.   As I drove past the gate, people whom I've known for years began shouting, 'Scab, scab'. Strikers were waving chains and steel pipes at me... It...it was extremely unsettling.

BRECHT   Maybe you ought to donate part of your salary to the workers who are out on strike.

LAUGHT.   I should probably do something.

BRECHT   It's the least you could do.

LAUGHT.   *(pause)* You're right... I'm...I'm going to write the union a check first thing in the morning.

BRECHT   I'll see you on Saturday.

LAUGHT.	You'll have to come over earlier next time. *(BRECHT shakes LAUGHTON'S hand.)*
BRECHT	*Gute Nacht. (BRECHT EXITS. LAUGHTON reads* Galileo Galilei *silently, periodically performs the dialogue's rhythm with his hands. ELSA eventually speaks.)*
ELSA	*(Offstage.)* Yoo-hoo, Charles...
LAUGHT.	Hello, love.
ELSA	*(ELSA ENTERS.)* I just saw Brecht pulling out of the driveway. He couldn't stay and say hello?
LAUGHT.	There's a curfew for 'enemy aliens'.
ELSA	'Enemy aliens'... You'd think Brecht and his German friends were about to attack Los Angeles with ray-guns, a fleet of flying saucers...
LAUGHT.	The government's just being cautious.
ELSA	It's this Flash-Gordon government I'm afraid of... Everyone with Japanese blood is being locked up in internment camps... Film scripts have to make it past the censor... You'd think the American government would welcome potential Fascists...
LAUGHT.	Brecht's far from being a Fascist.
ELSA	Oh, darling, the next time he comes over, would you take him out on the patio to smoke his cigars. It smells like a barn in here.
LAUGHT.	I don't smell anything.
ELSA	Your allergies must be acting up...
LAUGHT.	Brecht wants me to do *Galileo Galilei* on Broadway.
ELSA	Does he have a role for me?
LAUGHT.	Here, take a look. *(LAUGHTON hands ELSA the play.)* It's a wonderful play... Reminds me of Shakespeare, actually... And Brecht wants me to help him revise the script.
ELSA	Well, you've always wanted to write.
LAUGHT.	I haven't stepped on a stage in over ten years. And the play's so long. And I have film commitments... I'd be collaborating on the writing...

ELSA	I think you should do it. *(ELSA gets a bit amorous with LAUGHTON.)*
LAUGHT.	*(pause)* Perhaps I will.
ELSA	You must be so tired.
LAUGHT.	I'm...I'm still not confident with that long monologue...
ELSA	*(Amorous.)* Go over it in the morning.
LAUGHT.	It always sinks in better when I look it over just before going to sleep.
ELSA	Pour me a glass of wine.
LAUGHT.	I have to get to work.
ELSA	*(LAUGHTON is standing, looking at his film script. Pause.)* Sit down. *(ELSA pats the spot next to her on the couch.)*
LAUGHT.	I don't want to get distracted.
ELSA	I want you to make love to me, Charles.
LAUGHT.	When...when I come to bed later.
ELSA	You're always so much more fun on the couch.
LAUGHT.	I have to get these lines down.
ELSA	I'll wait up.
LAUGHT.	I might be a while.
ELSA	You can get up early and—
LAUGHT.	Why don't you just go to sleep.
ELSA	You just said you'd make love to me.
LAUGHT.	I...I will.
ELSA	You never wake me up to make love.
LAUGHT.	Good night. *(LAUGHTON kisses her.)*
ELSA	We never spend any time together.
LAUGHT.	We're together all day.
ELSA	We never spend any time together alone.
LAUGHT.	Well, when we're both shooting a film...getting up at five in the morning to be on the set...
ELSA	You're always shooting a film.
LAUGHT.	Fortunately.

ELSA	I guess we're *both* fortunate, aren't we? Now that we're working together and I get to play your adopted daughter all day.
LAUGHT.	I'll see you upstairs in a little while.
ELSA	*(pause)* Why weren't you on time for our parlor scene?
LAUGHT.	I...I had to take care of some business.
ELSA	What business?
LAUGHT.	The bank. I had to go to the bank.
ELSA	Well, Alex, the set decorator, saw you walking into the courthouse this afternoon. *(LAUGHTON goes over his lines.)* Were you at the courthouse?
LAUGHT.	Well...yes, that was one of my stops.
ELSA	For what?
LAUGHT.	I...I had to clear something up.
ELSA	Clear what up?
LAUGHT.	It was nothing, really.
ELSA	What?
LAUGHT.	It's taken care of.
ELSA	What's taken care of?
LAUGHT.	*(pause)* Somebody...somebody was trying to blackmail me...
ELSA	Why didn't you tell me?
LAUGHT.	I...I didn't want to worry you. But it's all cleared up now. *(LAUGHTON returns to his script.)*
ELSA	*(pause)* Who tried to blackmail you?
LAUGHT.	Well, it's...it's a bit complicated... But there was this lad...who was demanding money.
ELSA	For what?
LAUGHT.	Well... All right, you see... There...there was this lad, a struggling actor who was taking care of the crafts table. And I befriended him...by introducing him to my agent... But it became apparent that he didn't know how to act, so of course the agency couldn't work with him. And then—out of spite, I suppose—he said he was going to tell my agency that...that we had a tryst.

ELSA   You and this lad?

LAUGHT.   And then he said he was going to tell the newspapers. And all the studios. If I
            didn't give him money. And then he kept demanding more. And more.

ELSA   Why would the newspapers even believe him?

LAUGHT.   He said he had photographs. Which is absolutely ludicrous, of course, unless
            they were doctored. And when I told him I wasn't going to pay him anymore
            he...he threatened to hurt me... So I went to the police... And it's all been taken
            care of.

ELSA   Did the boy's accusations have any merit?

LAUGHT.   They're...accusations...

ELSA   So that's all there is to it?

LAUGHT.   *(pause)* Of course.

ELSA   Be honest with me, Charles.

LAUGHT.   Well...to be frank, as...as you may have already surmised...there...there have
            been times when...when I've had a...bit of a...homosexual streak...
            And...well....the lad and I did have some physical contact. But only once. And I
            promise it will not—

ELSA   It's all right, darling.

LAUGHT.   It will not happen again.

ELSA   I said it's all right!

LAUGHT.   I promise.

ELSA   I trust that this won't continue.

LAUGHT.   No...of course not.

ELSA   *(pause)* Did you have sex with him in this house?

LAUGHT.   Absolutely not.

ELSA   Have you *ever* had sex in the house?

LAUGHT.   Well...with you.

ELSA   With a man.

LAUGHT.   Well...

ELSA   Have you?

LAUGHT.   *(pause)* Once...

ELSA   Only once?

LAUGHT.   Yes.

ELSA   You're sure.

LAUGHT.   Just once.

ELSA   Where?

LAUGHT.   *(pause)* In the house.

ELSA   Where in the house?

LAUGHT.   *(pause)* On the couch.

ELSA   Our living room couch?

LAUGHT.   I'm sorry. I...I don't know what else to—

ELSA   Get rid of it.

LAUGHT.   What?

ELSA   Get rid of the couch.

LAUGHT.   *(pause)* What do I do with a couch?

ELSA   Just get it out of the house.

LAUGHT.   Okay... *(LAUGHTON looks at couch. Pause.)*

ELSA   Now.

LAUGHT.   A couch isn't the easiest thing to discard—

ELSA   Just get it out of here.

LAUGHT.   I'll...I'll put it out in the garage.

ELSA   I want it off the property.

LAUGHT.   *(pause)* How?

ELSA   I don't know... Take it to the Salvation Army.

LAUGHT.   I will not let this happen again.

ELSA   I don't want to talk about it.

LAUGHT.   I promise.

ELSA   Just get the couch out of my house. *(LAUGHTON begins dragging couch out of room. BLACKOUT.)*

(**Projection**: J. Edgar Hoover: We must beware of the threat from alien groups, foreign oppressions and noxious 'isms'...of writers who decry religion and argue that distance from God makes for happiness. Foreign interlopers, international swindlers, and espousers of alien philosophies cannot be permitted to hide behind masquerading fronts.)

SCENE FOUR

(BERLAU'S flat.)

(BERLAU is reading a communist tract, sipping water. BRECHT quietly ENTERS her apartment, puts keys in pocket.)

BRECHT   Hello, *Fräulein*. *(BRECHT hands BERLAU a red rose, kisses her.)*

BERLAU   Oh, how nice... And it's plastic.

BRECHT   They last longer.

BERLAU   Here. *(BERLAU hands BRECHT a newspaper clipping.)*

BRECHT   What's this?

BERLAU   An article about the Prague underground and the assassination of Heydrich the Hangman.

BRECHT   *(BERLAU hands article to BRECHT, who pockets it.)* Laughton might help me with the *Galileo Galilei* translation.

BERLAU   I'll just concentrate on *The Caucasian Chalk Circle*.

BRECHT   I'm going to need your assistance with *Galileo*.

BERLAU   Laughton has a much better command of English.

BRECHT   We'll still need someone to do the typing... Do you have a vase?

BERLAU   For a fake flower?

BRECHT   It doesn't really look fake.

BERLAU   Maybe you could stick it up your ass. *(BRECHT sticks flower in empty bottle. He smokes, takes a drink.)* I have some new ideas for the end of the play.

BRECHT   We're not working tonight. *(BRECHT drinks.)*

BERLAU	Since the Governor's Wife practically rips the child apart when she yanks him out of the circle, the judge declares her an unfit caretaker, even though she's the biological mother. So the judge awards the child to the peasant.
BRECHT	But the Governor's Wife still has her estates.
BERLAU	The judge can find her guilty of fraud.
BRECHT	And then he can confiscate all of her land.
BERLAU	But what becomes of it?
BRECHT	Playgrounds. For the children.
BERLAU	Perfect.
BRECHT	All we need now is a famous actress to play Grusha, like Luise Rainer...
BERLAU	She's too old for Grusha.
BRECHT	Not if she can get the play on Broadway.
BERLAU	It might be too radical.
BRECHT	I'm going to sell it as a harmless fairy tale... The bourgeoisie love fairy tales. *(BRECHT acts amorously towards BERLAU. She pulls away.)*
BERLAU	I'm still concerned about the play's politics.
BRECHT	Look... Aesthetically, the play's innovative... Its ideas are properly Marxist... *(BRECHT is physical with BERLAU.)* It's all there... So why don't we fuck? *(BERLAU massages BRECHT'S neck. BRECHT plays with her hair.)*
BERLAU	We have to write out the ending.
BRECHT	We'll write it tomorrow night.
BERLAU	I don't want to wait that long.
BRECHT	Tomorrow afternoon... No, that won't work. Helly needs me around the house.
BERLAU	For what?
BRECHT	The children.
BERLAU	So now you're going to take more time away from me. *(BERLAU straddles him.)*
BRECHT	*(pause)* I don't want to.
BERLAU	You shouldn't.
BRECHT	I *do* have a family.

BERLAU	And what do I have?
BRECHT	*(pause)* Freedom... From children running around the house.
BERLAU	That's what I want.
BRECHT	God knows there are going to be enough orphans after the war.
BERLAU	My baby would have been twenty-two years old by now. About the same age as Frank. But I didn't need a child then.
BRECHT	I should have made sure Frank got out.
BERLAU	He has his mother.
BRECHT	Last I heard, Frank was being sent from relative to relative. My relatives, his mother's...
BERLAU	I want my own baby.
BRECHT	Wait till we get back to Germany.
BERLAU	I'm thirty-seven years old.
BRECHT	Ruth, look...once I start selling my work here, I'll be in a better position—
BERLAU	I need you around more Brecht.
BRECHT	I'll try to come by more often—
BERLAU	Without a wife to return to all the time. And I need a child sleeping in the other room as I work on my novel...
BRECHT	Let's just focus on writing out the ending.
BERLAU	*(pause)* I can't.
BRECHT	It was your idea to write tonight in the first place.
BERLAU	I'm going out for a walk. *(BERLAU begins to EXIT.)*
BRECHT	Rainer wants a copy of *The Caucasian Chalk Circle* by the end of the week.
BERLAU	You can use my typewriter.
BRECHT	We'll work on it when you return.
BERLAU	When I come back, I'm going to sleep.
BRECHT	We can finish it in the morning...
BERLAU	*(pause)* I'm leaving for New York tomorrow.
BRECHT	What?
BERLAU	I'm attending a conference there, on anti-Fascist resistance in Denmark.

BRECHT	When are you coming back?
BERLAU	I'm not sure.
BRECHT	Well, the conference has to end sometime.
BERLAU	I also have a job interview.
BRECHT	In New York?
BERLAU	I need to work, Brecht.
BRECHT	I'm paying your rent.
BERLAU	I need to do my own work.
BRECHT	It's *our* work.
BERLAU	I need to do work that's not for you.
BRECHT	Ruth, we've been collaborating on this for almost two years.
BERLAU	You know how to write.
BRECHT	I'm too used to members of the collective helping with the writing.
BERLAU	And fucking.
BRECHT	Primarily writing—
BERLAU	Writing and fucking. Fucking and writing. Fucking fucking, writing writing—
BRECHT	Right now I just want to finish the fucking play.
BERLAU	You want me to keep giving...and waiting... As you get your work published, produced—
BRECHT	At the very least, we're both going to make some money once the play gets to Broadway—
BERLAU	Do you think that's why I've been spending all this time with you? For money?
BRECHT	Of course there's much more than—
BERLAU	All your collaborators work for free anyway. Except for Kurt Weill, who's a man, so you can't fuck him like you fucked Margarete and Elisabeth and me and your fucking wife, God bless her... Weill could do something you couldn't take credit for, compose music, so you had to pay him... But me, you just keep fucking—and I let you—because I believe in what Brecht's trying to accomplish...
BRECHT	What *we're* trying to accomplish.

BERLAU   Why don't you put my name on *The Caucasian Chalk Circle* instead of yours?

BRECHT   Well...bourgeois publishers don't understand the notion of collective authorship yet...and my name's more recognizable. But we're splitting—

BERLAU   I must be a goddamn idiot... You storm into Copenhagen with your entourage and I give up my theatre, my writing career—which was just beginning to flourish—to work for Brecht... I walk away from my marriage to a physician, a potential family, so I can fuck Brecht without feeling guilty... And I've continued to write for Brecht, to sleep with Brecht, for nine fucking years... And still...I don't have a play or a child I can call my own.

BRECHT   Ruth, you're the most important person in my life.

BERLAU   I'm going out for a walk. And then I'm coming home, and going to bed. And then I'm going to wake up, pack my suitcase, take a taxi to Union Station, and leave for New York.

BRECHT   We finally have a chance to get a play produced on Broadway.

BERLAU   You have your friend Laughton to work with on *Galileo*.

BRECHT   I don't even know if he's interested.

BERLAU   At least he understands English. *(BERLAU EXITS, followed by BRECHT.. Note: while she is in New York, the audience may often see BERLAU, at times, on a video monitor. Phone eventually rings.)*

(Projection:
Ornate mansions shielded by electric gates
Stand minutes from decrepit sidewalks
Full of cardboard boxes
Housing families of four.
Yet the worry of losing it all
Affects those with live-in butlers
As much as the dwellers of streets.
—bb)

SCENE FIVE

(BRECHT'S front yard.)

BRECHT   *(BRECHT ENTERS with phone.)* Hello... Hallo, Luise. *Guten Tag...* Yes, yes... I know you're leaving on a USO tour... I just have to finish proofreading the script... Who? Leventhal? Of course, if there's a Broadway producer involved I'm going to need some money up front... At least fifteen hundred... Well, see what you can do... Yes, yes, the play's being translated... *Danke sehr. (BRECHT hangs up phone.)*

(**Projection**: FBI file on R. Berlau: On June 13 a 120 day mail cover was placed on Ruth Berlau at 123 East 57 Street, New York.)

BRECHT   Why do I have to put up with this crap? I feel as if I've been removed from civilization... This...this is Guatemala, posing as a modern city... I feel like Gandhi at Mardi Gras, Stalin on a ferris wheel...

ANGEL   Hey, Brecht...

BRECHT   A polar bear in the South Seas... Hell...

ANGEL   Brecht!

BRECHT   What?

ANGEL   You been to Mexican Town, yet, where the kids play on the sides of the dirt roads all day, runnin' through the muddy sewage in their barefeet... To *las cantinas* on Central Avenue? To skid row?

BRECHT   I'm certainly aware of those places.

ANGEL   You been to 'em? To the dirt-floored brothels up in Boyle Heights?

BRECHT   I, uh...went to a strip joint in Malibu.

ANGEL   When you gonna go see where the other half lives?

BRECHT   I've driven all over the city.

ANGEL   You ever stop and get out of the car anywhere except Santa Monica and Pacific Palisades?

BRECHT   I observe, I read...

ANGEL	Down here it's always cool breezes, ocean.
BRECHT	Helps make hell bearable for me.
ANGEL	You don't know what hell is till you've stood in the fire.
BRECHT	The fire's gotta be extinguished.
ANGEL	By you?
BRECHT	Well, I can't do it myself.
ANGEL	You can't put the fire out at all. Nobody can. Until they can feel the heat...

(ANGEL EXITS, BRECHT tries to puff on cigar; it's out.)

BRECHT	Helly...do you have any matches in there? *(BRECHT EXITS.)*

(**Projection**: at times, when motoring past the majestic gardens of belaire or pasadena, i actually believe i'm among 'nature'. but then i'm jolted back to reality as i begin to calculate the value of the land, the imported palm trees, the cost of irrigating it all through millions of miles of pipes connected to distant lakes. one is always calculating the value of people here, too. —bb)

SCENE SIX

(BRECHT'S front yard, two weeks later.)

(LAUGHTON knocks on BRECHT'S front door one last time, looks at watch, walks away from door. TOM ENTERS.)

TOM	Hi, there.
LAUGHT.	Good evening.
TOM	You know, you look familiar.
LAUGHT.	I have that sort of face. *(LAUGHTON walks towards street.)*
TOM	You're...you're a movie star, aren't you?
LAUGHT.	Well...
TOM	The...*The Hunchback of Notre Dame....* You're the Hunchback of Notre Dame.
LAUGHT.	Well, that was one of my roles...
TOM	You were hilarious.
LAUGHT.	*(pause)* Thank you. *(LAUGHTON walks.)*

TOM   Hey, are you looking for Breath?

LAUGHT.   Brecht.

TOM   *(Periodically, LAUGHTON wipes sweat from his face, neck with a*

             handkerchief.) I, uh...I saw you knocking on his door.

LAUGHT.   Are you a friend of his?

TOM   Yes... We're very good friends, actually...

LAUGHT.   I was supposed to meet him here.

TOM   My name's Tom by the way. *(TOM offers his hand.)*

LAUGHT.   Charles. *(They shake hands.)*

TOM   You know Breath pretty well?

LAUGHT.   Brecht... We're working together on a project.

TOM   You're acting in one of his plays?

LAUGHT.   At the moment, I'm helping him to revise a play.

TOM   What about?

LAUGHT.   Galileo.

TOM   Oh, the scientist.

LAUGHT.   Well, it was nice to have met you. *(LAUGHTON begins to leave.)*

TOM   I'm a writer, too, you know.

LAUGHT.   Good luck to you. *(LAUGHTON goes to leave.)*

TOM   Breath often asks me for advice.

LAUGHT.   Tell him Charles Laughton dropped by.

TOM   Where are you from?

LAUGHT.   Pacific Palisades.

TOM   No, I mean what country.

LAUGHT.   England. *(LAUGHTON looks at watch, seems inclined to leave.)*

TOM   I'm sure he'll be right back.

LAUGHT.   He told you this?

TOM   He has curfew. *(TOM looks at his watch.)* Which means that if he's not back

             here within...twenty-two minutes, a neighbor could report him to the police.

LAUGHT.   Why would a neighbor do that?

TOM   Well, I'm not sure that anyone would...

LAUGHT.   I would hope not.

TOM   But you never know.

LAUGHT.   Well, I'm not about to stand out here waiting for twenty minutes.

TOM   Why don't you come wait at my place?

LAUGHT.   I'm just going to be heading home.

TOM   I'll make some iced-tea.

LAUGHT.   Oh, I don't want to impose.

TOM   Impose? I'd be honored.

LAUGHT.   I don't want to disrupt the household.

TOM   I *am* the household. Just me and the cat.

LAUGHT.   Well, I... *(LAUGHTON is sweating profusely.)*

TOM   I'd really like to hear about this play you're working on.

LAUGHT.   It's Brecht's play, actually.

TOM   Galileo was against the Bible, wasn't he?

LAUGHT.   I'm more interested in the play's theatrical aspects. *(LAUGHTON is ready to
             leave. TOM glances at his watch.)*

TOM   You know, every movie I've ever seen you in, your character always stands out.

LAUGHT.   Well, I try...

TOM   Even when you're playing a minor role...or some buffoon that most established
             actors wouldn't touch with a ten-foot pole.

LAUGHT.   Thank you. *(LAUGHTON begins to EXIT.)*

TOM   You have to stop in for a cold drink.

LAUGHT.   Well...

TOM   My kitchen table's right next to the window. You'll see Breath's car as soon as
             he pulls in.

LAUGHT.   Well, perhaps I can stop in for a couple of minutes. *(They start walking towards
             house.)*

TOM   Are you a bachelor?

LAUGHT.   No... Not exactly.

TOM   'Not exactly'? *(TOM smiles.)*

LAUGHT.   I'm parched.

TOM   If you'd like something stronger, I also have excellent Scotch...Dom Perignon...

LAUGHT.   Scotch would be fine.

TOM   You know, I've always wanted to get into acting.

LAUGHT.   Well, you have the proper looks.

TOM   You think so?

LAUGHT.   You'll just need to work on technique.

TOM   Maybe you can give me some advice. *(TOM puts his arm on LAUGHTON'S shoulder, accompanies him towards his house.)*

LAUGHT.   I'd be glad to. *(EXEUNT. The audience hears a car pull up, a car door open and close. BRECHT ENTERS, gets mail, looks at watch.)*

BRECHT   I hope Laughton shows up. *(BRECHT sorts through mail.)* 'Opened by mistake'. 'Opened by mistake'. Leventhal...that's the producer... *(BRECHT opens letter, pulls out check.)* Seven hundred and fifty dollars?... He was supposed to send me fifteen hundred... Fucking reptile... *(BRECHT continues sorting through mail.)* 'Opened by mistake'. This one's taped up... I thought only the *Gestapo* was reading my mail... New York... *(BRECHT reads the lines within the quotation marks to himself as BERLAU, in a white nightgown, speaks them from another part of the stage.)*

BERLAU   Dear Brecht, I am content. With you. And I thank you. Thank you. Of course, I worry from time to time, but that is mostly because I'm afraid that you won't remain faithful... *(BRECHT chuckles.)* I assumed that you would be saying to yourself, 'I'm glad she moved to New York, a good riddance', and then you told me to hurry back to California... I'm glad that you're so strict with me. Enclosed is the German version of *Caucasian Chalk Circle*... As you requested, Auden's begun the translation work. Yours always, Ruth. *(Here and elsewhere, BERLAU might occasionally look up to the sky with a small telescope.)*

BRECHT   *(Phone rings. BRECHT answers it.)* Yes, Luise... I was just about to bring it over... In German... Yes, I know I promised the English version two weeks ago... I can get it to you by Friday. But I need the money from Leventhal... Well, he hasn't sent it yet... *Auf Wiedersehen.*

(**Projection**: J. Edgar Hoover: Today vile and vicious forces are seeking to tear America asunder, killing freedom, ravishing justice, and destroying liberty... The subversive group, those termites of discontent, can be neutralized only by a holy war.)

SCENE SEVEN

(BRECHT'S front yard, next morning.)

(It's early morning, birds are chirping. BRECHT sits with a cup of coffee. He wears slippers, a silk robe over his clothes. He's smoking a cigar and writing quickly, with great intensity. After a successful onrush of writing, BRECHT pauses, speaks.)

BRECHT   This is just what I need... To get outside first thing in the morning...while the day's still fresh... While the bird's are chirping and everything's placid, peaceful... *(BRECHT writes for a while, smiles.)* This is going to be my best day of writing since arriving in California... *(BRECHT writes for a few more seconds and then a gasoline lawnmower starts up.) Vas ist denn los... (ANGEL ENTERS with lawnmower.)* Hey... Hey... *(ANGEL neither sees nor hears BRECHT. BRECHT walks over to him.)* What the hell are you doing?

ANGEL   *(ANGEL smiles, nods head, continues mowing.) Sí.*

BRECHT   *(BRECHT stops him.).* Hey... It's seven o'clock in the morning... I need you to stop.

ANGEL   *Un minuto. (ANGEL turns off lawnmower.)* What?

BRECHT   It's seven a.m.

ANGEL   I wake you up?

BRECHT   I'm trying to get some work done, damn it.

ANGEL   Me too.

BRECHT   I just thought I'd have a bit more time before I had to start listening to the—

ANGEL   I'll be done in ten minutes. *(ANGEL is about to start lawnmower again.)*

BRECHT   Maybe you can begin by doing— *(Lawnmower starts.)* Hey. Hey!!! Turn that thing off!

ANGEL   The more of those cheap cigars people buy, the more jobs get replaced by machines.

BRECHT   You use a machine to cut grass, don't you? And it enables you to make more money.

ANGEL   It enables *you* to get your lawn cut more cheaply, no?

BRECHT   If I can't sell a play soon, I might have to start mowing lawns with you.

ANGEL   I don't think you could do it.

BRECHT   What?

ANGEL   Cut grass. *(ANGEL readies the tools of his trade.)*

BRECHT   Anybody could cut grass.

ANGEL   When's the last time you did any manual labor? *(ANGEL works.)*

BRECHT   Well, I, uh... *(ANGEL EXITS, continues to operate manual hedge clippers. BRECHT tries to write. Eventually, ELSA ENTERS.)*

ELSA   Good morning.

BRECHT   Hello, Mrs. Laughton.

ELSA   Oh...Elsa. *(ELSA sniffs the air, intermittently, throughout scene.)*

BRECHT   Elsa...

ELSA   Have you seen Charles at all?

BRECHT   No.

ELSA   He said he was going over to your house last night.

BRECHT   He never showed up.

ELSA   What's that odor?

BRECHT   *(BRECHT takes a whiff of the air.).* I don't smell anything.

ELSA   We're supposed to be on the set in a couple of hours and I have absolutely no idea where he is.

BRECHT   I'm sure he'll show up there.

ELSA   He never came home last night.

BRECHT	You know how Charles likes to talk... He probably stopped at someone's house, had a few drinks, and before he knew it, he was laid out on their couch.
ELSA	What couch?
BRECHT	A friend's couch.
ELSA	What was he doing on a couch?
BRECHT	What do people usually do on a couch?
ELSA	Well...that depends.
BRECHT	He was probably sleeping.
ELSA	He never stays out all night.
BRECHT	He's probably trying to call you right now.
ELSA	I could hardly sleep, I was so worried.
BRECHT	Let me get you a cup of coffee.
ELSA	Is your wife awake?
BRECHT	She's up in Santa Barbara with the children.
ELSA	Where's your mistress?
BRECHT	I don't have a mistress.
ELSA	That Danish actress I always see you with...
BRECHT	She's just an assistant. And she lives in New York now.
ELSA	Charles has been so energized over the past few weeks from working with you on *Galileo Galilei*.
BRECHT	Your husband's making the play stronger. He's been emphasizing Galileo's polarities. He's always thinking, yet has a weakness for things of the flesh... He's highly intelligent, yet also a coward...
ELSA	Charles must be just perfect.
BRECHT	Absolutely.
ELSA	Too bad there isn't a role for me.
BRECHT	You can play Galileo's servant.
ELSA	She's subservient to a man.

BRECHT *(ELSA gets matches, eventually lights BRECHT'S cigar.)* If you utilize the techniques of my epic theatre, you'll be able to perform patriarchal subservience while simultaneously critiquing it.

ELSA Galileo's servant has three lines.

BRECHT Well...I have plenty of strong women in other plays. Like Mother Courage, which I think you'd be perfect for.

ELSA You've never even seen me perform.

BRECHT I saw you at the Turnabout Theatre.

ELSA You saw that?

BRECHT Yes. And I was very impressed... You were a performer up there, not some method actor trying to hide behind the fourth wall.

ELSA Well, I began my career as a cabaret artist in London.

BRECHT You have to play Mother Courage... She travels from battle to battle selling whatever's at hand. To soldiers. But she's always in charge... And she's also a pacifist, a feminist. And she's a performer...she sings. You'd fit the role perfectly.

ELSA I'd just about given up hope of ever finding a decent part out here.

BRECHT Why don't you come in for a cup of coffee and we'll, uh...discuss the play.

ELSA Oh, I have to go find Charles.

BRECHT Charles is a big boy... He's fine.

ELSA I hope so.

BRECHT Let me show you the house.

ELSA Oh, I wouldn't want your wife to get the wrong idea.

BRECHT My wife let's me do what I please...as long as I keep her happy.

ELSA *(Looks at watch.)* I should probably get to the studio.

BRECHT You have two hours.

ELSA I like to relax in my dressing room before going to work.

BRECHT With all those protestors shouting outside the gate?

ELSA There really aren't that many.

BRECHT Don't Hollywood actors have any conscience?

57

ELSA   If you have a conscience, you don't act in Hollywood.

BRECHT   I love your sweater. *(BRECHT fingers the sweater.)*

ELSA   Charles gave it to me.

BRECHT   I never realized your eyes had such color.

ELSA   They get puffy when I haven't slept.

BRECHT   They're so clear.

ELSA   There's that smell again...

BRECHT   Must be the neighbor's garbage...

ELSA   Otherwise, it's...it's quite pleasant out here...

BRECHT   Nice and quiet...

ELSA   Yes, and I...I appreciate the serenity... After being up all night worrying, it's exactly what I need right now. *(BRECHT puts his arm around ELSA. Lawnmower starts up offstage. ELSA jumps.)*

BRECHT   *(Hollering.)* Let's go inside! *(ANGEL ENTERS, walks by with lawnmower. BRECHT ENTERS house with ELSA, with his arm around her. LAUGHTON ENTERS, looking as if he'd been up late drinking.)*

LAUGHT.   What the hell... *(He tries to fix his hair, tie, etc., stares at car in BRECHT'S driveway.)* What... What's Elsa's car doing there... *(Looks at watch, EXITS.)* And that wanker told me his wife was going to be out of town... *(LAUGHTON EXITS, BERLAU opens letter.)*

(**Projection**: FBI file on R. Berlau: Ruth Berlau has been said to be critical of United States' policy and to advocate communism in this country.)

(**Projection**: FBI file on B. Brecht: Subject's writings...advocate overthrow of Capitalism, establishment of Communist State, and use of sabotage by labor to attain its ends.)

SCENE EIGHT

(New York/Los Angeles.)

BRECHT   *(offstage)* *(BERLAU reads letter silently as BRECHT speaks its words.)* Dear Ruth, I'm forever thinking of you and I entreat you, my love, to remain constant during these darkest of days. I've received an advance...but the criminal producer paid me only half of the agreed upon amount. As promised, I am sending you a check for half of what I received, two hundred dollars. Love always, bb.

                p.s. a grayish mist drifted in from the Pacific last night, so I couldn't see the stars. but I was sure you were gazing skyward, so, in a way, I was there with you...

BERLAU   *(BERLAU writes a bit, reads.)* The person I love...isn't here, although I can feel his weight... But I love. I'm in love. I am jealous...in love...and the...the devils won't let go of me... I'm...I'm so full of jealousy and love that the devil's fire is scorching my body... *(BERLAU'S phone rings.)* Yet the pleasure of lust, with you, far outweighs any pain. *(BERLAU answers phone.)* Yes? *(BRECHT ENTERS with phone.)*

BRECHT   Hello, darling.

BERLAU   Brecht.

BRECHT   What's that clicking sound?

BERLAU   I don't hear anything.

BRECHT   No?

BERLAU   I was just thinking about you.

BRECHT   Is anyone there?

BERLAU   No... But my crotch has been burning for you...

BRECHT   Good.

BERLAU   It keeps getting hotter...and hotter...

BRECHT   Are you wearing your white nightgown?

BERLAU   Yes, but if you don't get here soon it's going to be nothing but ashes.

BRECHT	Just wait for me to put out the fire.
BERLAU	When are you coming to New York?
BRECHT	As soon as I get some money.
BERLAU	You have the money from Rainer.
BRECHT	Not after I pay the mortgage.
BERLAU	Once you get the rest of the advance, you'll have to hop on a plane.
BRECHT	Her producer friend needs to see the script first.
BERLAU	You have the script.
BRECHT	He needs to see it in English. What's going on with Auden?
BERLAU	I haven't been able to find him lately.
BRECHT	If I don't get the English translation within the next few days, the entire deal's going to fall apart...
BERLAU	I keep calling him. He's never in.
BRECHT	Go to Auden's apartment. As soon as we get off the phone.
BERLAU	I'm too tired.
BRECHT	Tired? It's Sunday.
BERLAU	It's ten o'clock at night here.
BRECHT	What have you been doing all day?
BERLAU	I...I went to a shower.
BRECHT	You have a friend who's getting married?
BERLAU	I went to a baby shower.
BRECHT	I thought you didn't have any friends there?
BERLAU	It was all co-workers.
BRECHT	You shouldn't be wasting your time at work-related functions unless you're getting paid.
BERLAU	*(pause)* The shower was for me.
BRECHT	What?
BERLAU	I'm seven weeks pregnant.
BRECHT	*(pause)* So who's the lucky man?
BERLAU	What kind of question is that?

BRECHT	I'm sure there are plenty of doctors in New York who can take care of it for you.
BERLAU	This might be our only opportunity.
BRECHT	We can't have a baby now.
BERLAU	I don't have any choice.
BRECHT	Of course you have a choice, Ruth. There are—
BERLAU	*(BERLAU puts down phone.)*. I'm having the baby. *(BRECHT puts down phone. They speak directly to each other.)*
BRECHT	Have you seen a doctor yet?
BERLAU	I went to a clinic.
BRECHT	Clinical examinations aren't very accurate.
BERLAU	I went to two clinics. I got the same result each time.
BRECHT	You have to go see a regular doctor. In an office.
BERLAU	Are you going to pay for it?
BRECHT	I'll be sending you another check if Auden ever finishes the damn translation.
BERLAU	I have to see a doctor regularly.
BRECHT	Go to the clinic.
BERLAU	They don't provide prenatal care there.
BRECHT	You'll be fine.
BERLAU	How am I supposed to make sure that the baby's okay?
BRECHT	You're making more money than me.
BERLAU	*(pause)* I'm not making anything.
BRECHT	What?
BERLAU	I was fired from my job.
BRECHT	For what?
BERLAU	Well...according to my boss, I was fighting against the wrong side in Spain.
BRECHT	You were fighting against fascism...
BERLAU	My friend thinks I was fired for getting pregnant out of wedlock...
BRECHT	You haven't told anyone else...
BERLAU	No.
BRECHT	I want you to keep it that way.

BERLAU   How am I going to pay the rent?

BRECHT   Find Auden and get me the translation.

BERLAU   I don't even know if he's in New York.

BRECHT   Rainer wanted the translation by today.

BERLAU   I need your support.

BRECHT   I'll...I'll do whatever I can, Ruth. Okay?

BERLAU   I love you... You know, having a baby together isn't the worst thing that could happen to us.

BRECHT   I love the idea of having a baby with you.

BERLAU   Really?

BRECHT   As long as he doesn't look like me.

BERLAU   He'll probably come out with a cigar in his mouth.

BRECHT   Why don't we make him wait a couple of years?

BERLAU   I love you.

BRECHT   You, too, darling. *(BRECHT turns away, speaks into phone.)* Now find Auden and send me the script. *(They hang up. BERLAU eventually writes, intermittently looks at and caresses her stomach. BRECHT moves to his front yard.)* Jesus Christ. *(BRECHT hangs up phone, tries to write. ANGEL ENTERS with gardening tools.)*

ANGEL   I made this for you. *(ANGEL gives BRECHT a cigar.)*

BRECHT   Here. *(BRECHT attempts to give ANGEL a quarter.)*

ANGEL   The tobacco doesn't belong to me.

BRECHT   You made this, right?

ANGEL   Yes.

BRECHT   Just take it.

ANGEL   To my ancestors, the Tay-ahno, cigars were always for healing, gifts... But then Columbus 'discovered' cigars...and the tobacco's smoke, which—to us—had always represented freedom, became the devil's spirit. Its fire, which freed the spirit, became hell. Eventually, though, aristocrats realized that they could sell cigars for a profit. Thus, cigars were no longer evil. So while Indians were being burned at the stake, cigars were burning in the mouths of white men.

BRECHT   So I'm complicit in all that...

ANGEL   (pause) As long as you continue to consume the present without recognizing the past. *(ANGEL EXITS. BRECHT holds up the cigar.)*

BRECHT   This is only a fucking cigar. *(BRECHT'S phone rings; he answers. ANGEL may softly speak the lines of the following projection as BRECHT speaks on the phone.)*

(**Projection**: the desire to examine on the stage, in a critical light, issues of pressing concern to the nation is viewed as completely ridiculous here. for a writer to 'win' his spectators must lose. —bb)

BRECHT   Hello... Hello, Luise. *Wie geht es Ihnen?* Yes, I know you only have the German version, but I... What... You expected Grusha to be more sympathetic?... Then the audience will be more concerned with Grusha than the play's politics... Yes, I know people will be buying tickets because they want to see you... I also thought Auden would be finished by now... Look...if you can just give me another week or so... What? I can't believe this... You told me we had a deal...

BERLAU   *(BERLAU speaks as if possessed.)* The roof collapses... And I can feel flames...erupting all over my body...

BRECHT   To tell you the truth, Luise, perhaps it's just as well... Because you're much too old for the part anyway. *(BLACKOUT on BRECHT. SPOTLIGHT on BERLAU.)*

BERLAU   Oddly...my pubic hair is the only thing that burns... Unable to put out the fire with my hands, I attempt to douse the flames...with the water of my womb. *(BLACKOUT).*

ACT II

SCENE NINE

(BRECHT'S front yard.)

ANGEL   *(BRECHT ENTERS.)* Hey, Brecht... Brecht!

BRECHT   I'm on my way somewhere.

ANGEL   You keep goin' on and on complaining about consumerism...

BRECHT   I can't help it. I'm swimming in it here. And if I don't start kicking harder it's going to swallow me up.

ANGEL   When are you gonna start doing something to change all this?

BRECHT   That's what my epic theatre's all about. It encourages the audience to participate, actively, in radically changing the world.

ANGEL   So you think it's enough to use a typewriter, or the stage, to create revolution.

BRECHT   Well, that's my only means at the moment.

ANGEL   An underground group I belong to has a stockpile of weapons outside Havana. Plans for attacking government strongholds.

BRECHT   I thought your Communist Party was supporting the Cuban government.

ANGEL   They are. Because it's benefitting the people at the top of the Communist Party. But my group, we're going to transform the structure of society by attacking hierarchy. At all levels. And I'd like you to accompany us.

BRECHT   Well, I'll do what I can...

ANGEL   I'll give you your own machine gun.

BRECHT   Well...thanks... But, uh...once the war ends, I have to carry on the battle against fascism in Germany.

ANGEL   You can come to Cuba with me *before* the war's over.

BRECHT   I'd like to, but I, uh...I have my children...

ANGEL   I have a young daughter. And I'd like to be with her. But it's unsafe for me to be in my country right now. Although I'll have to go back, eventually.

BRECHT   Sometimes it's best to operate from afar. *(BRECHT looks at his watch.)* And I,

uh, have an appointment to get to.

(**Projection**: turning a quick buck is seen as a noble act. you're courteous only to the extent
that it will enhance your deal. you sell your snot, if you can, to the handkerchief. —bb)

SCENE TEN

(LANG'S office.)

BRECHT   There's a radical pig farmer from Kentucky. He could be played by Peter Lorre.

LANG   Peter Lorre's all fucked up.

BRECHT   He did some brilliant stage work for me over in—

LANG   Lorre doesn't even leave his house anymore. He sits around all day strung out

on morphine.

BRECHT   I'm sorry to hear that—

LANG   Look, Brecht, I know you're having difficulties here. But the fucking studio's

got me working my ass off right now and I'm not going to be able to consider

any more stories until next year.

BRECHT   Lang, I've got children to feed.

LANG   What is it now, four, five?

BRECHT   I have two that are with me here. And a wife.

LANG   And how many mistresses?

BRECHT   The mistress is in New York.

LANG   So now you have a place to visit.

BRECHT   What, exactly, are you looking for in a screenplay?

LANG   At the moment, the topic everyone's interested in is war.

BRECHT   Well, I have *Mother Courage*.

LANG   World War II. It's huge right now.

BRECHT   Well, with half the world's countries sucked into it—

LANG   It's huge for the film business.

BRECHT   In Hollywood.

LANG	The film business *is* Hollywood.
BRECHT	As long as Japan doesn't start dropping bombs on Los Angeles.
LANG	That's exactly the sort of threat that's selling movie tickets right now. Which is why the studios are rushing to get war films out before the fervor dies down. As we speak they're filming *Spy Smashers*, *Yellow Peril*, *V. is for Victory*... A mega-musical, *I'll Take Manila*.
BRECHT	The Japanese have just about taken Manila.
LANG	So the studio can change the title to...to...I don't know...*I'll Take Tahiti*... Who gives a damn? As long as the audience gets to see palm trees, tanks, machine-gun fire... *(LANG looks at his watch.)*
BRECHT	How about this... Someone from the Czech resistance ambushes the deputy chief of the *Gestapo*, Heydrich the Hangman.
LANG	The *Gestapo's* very popular right now... But Americans could care less about a Czechoslovakian hero.
BRECHT	We'll include American marines.
LANG	Or we can keep the movie all Czechs and Germans, but have the Czechs speak with American accents, so then, as far as the audience is concerned, the Czechs are American.
BRECHT	Heydrich's assassin appears at a clandestine meeting of the Prague underground, where he gives a speech against imperialism.
LANG	Hollywood wants to colonize foreign markets.
BRECHT	So the speech can emphasize the absurdity of war.
LANG	Violence and patriotism sell tickets.
BRECHT	We can have flashbacks to concentration camps full of shirtless, emaciated Jews splitting boulders.
LANG	Impossible.
BRECHT	It's reality.
LANG	Film creates its own reality.
BRECHT	But it must also be connected to the world.

LANG	Look, Brecht, if this film is going to get made, it cannot depict Nazi atrocities against Jews.
BRECHT	You're Jewish for Christ's sake.
LANG	Brecht, you're in America... So stick with what the American government wants people to see and you can make a lot of money...
BRECHT	*(pause)* We'll call the film *Trust the People*.
LANG	Too socialist.
BRECHT	Why don't we call it *Trust Capital: Why Fascism's Good for Business*?
LANG	Do you want to work in Hollywood or not?
BRECHT	I have to.
LANG	I'm going to try to sell this idea of yours.
BRECHT	How much is it going to pay?
LANG	Let me pitch it to the studio first, and then we'll talk. *(Looks at watch, stands.)* And I'm running late for a luncheon meeting with Shirley Temple and Lassie... Jesus Christ, who are they gonna ask me to work with next, a tap-dancing cocker spaniel? *(LANG EXITS. BRECHT EXITS into hall. ELSA ENTERS.)*
ELSA	Brecht.
BRECHT	Hello, darling.
ELSA	I told you not to visit me here.
BRECHT	I was just pitching a film script. But I'm glad I ran into you. *(BRECHT pulls her close. She moves away.)*
ELSA	No one can see us together.
BRECHT	Where's your husband?
ELSA	We just started working together on a new film.
BRECHT	Has Charles been a good boy lately?
ELSA	I could care less what Charles does in his free time.
BRECHT	Are you busy?
ELSA	I have about half an hour.
BRECHT	Step into my office.
ELSA	You don't have an office.

BRECHT	It's right there.
ELSA	That's Fritz Lang's.
BRECHT	He said I could use it. *(BRECHT puts his arm around her. ELSA sniffs the air.)*
ELSA	There's that smell again.
BRECHT	I'll light a cigar.
ELSA	Not one of those cheap cigars...
BRECHT	Lang has top-shelf cigars in the office. Would you like one?
ELSA	What if Lang walks in?
BRECHT	He just went to lunch.
ELSA	He might come back early.
BRECHT	Don't worry. He's an old friend... C'mon, let's go inside. *(ELSA sniffs the air. BRECHT gently pushes ELSA towards office, which she ENTERS.)*
ELSA	*(Offstage.)* This office is quite lovely... *(LAUGHTON ENTERS.)*
LAUGHT.	Brecht.
BRECHT	*(To ELSA, who is in office.)* I'll be right there. *(BRECHT shuts LANG'S door, remains in hall.)* Hello, my friend.
LAUGHT.	You can't get enough, can you?
BRECHT	Well, I—
LAUGHT.	So now you show up at the studio.
BRECHT	Well, I'm certainly free to go elsewhere.
LAUGHT.	You better be careful where you hang your hat, pal.
BRECHT	I never realized you had an exclusive contract.
LAUGHT.	You're lucky we have an agreement.
BRECHT	What agreement?
LAUGHT.	Between me and my wife.
BRECHT	I'm talking about *Galileo*... It's not the only project I'm working on at the moment, thank God. I just pitched a film to Fritz Lang.
LAUGHT.	*(pause)* That's why you're here?
BRECHT	Why else would I be here?
LAUGHT.	Well, I...I drove by your house this morning.

BRECHT	For what?
LAUGHT.	On my way to the studio.
BRECHT	I don't live anywhere near the studio.
LAUGHT.	Well, I...I went by anyway, thinking I might catch you outside.
BRECHT	What time did you drive by?
LAUGHT.	About 7:15.
BRECHT	How could you miss me?
LAUGHT.	I drove right by and—
BRECHT	I was sitting on the front step.
LAUGHT.	No you weren't.
BRECHT	You should have honked.
LAUGHT.	My wife's car was in your driveway.
BRECHT	What car?
LAUGHT.	A red Cadillac. With whitewall tires.
BRECHT	Oh, that's the gardener's.
LAUGHT.	Why would a gardener drive a new Cadillac?
BRECHT	Why not? He's entitled.
LAUGHT.	They don't make enough money.
BRECHT	How would you know what gardeners make?
LAUGHT.	Well, I don't, but—
BRECHT	He works in Beverly Hills...
LAUGHT.	Well, still, he—
BRECHT	I pay him top dollar.
LAUGHT.	I never saw a new Cadillac carrying lawnmowers.
BRECHT	Have you ever seen a Cadillac's trunk? You can fit five lawnmowers and a small church choir back there.
LAUGHT.	It looked exactly like my wife's car.
BRECHT	There must be ten thousand people driving red Cadillacs around here.
LAUGHT.	You didn't see my wife this morning?
BRECHT	No. Of course not.

LAUGHT.	I'm surprised you're here.
BRECHT	Well...my family has to eat.
LAUGHT.	So that justifies crossing a picket line?
BRECHT	I didn't see any picket line.
LAUGHT.	It's right outside the front gate.
BRECHT	I came in through the back lot with Fritz Lang.
LAUGHT.	Well, there's still a strike going on.
BRECHT	But I didn't see it, so, I, uh...I assumed it was settled.
LAUGHT.	I guess you don't need me anymore for *Galileo*.
BRECHT	What are you talking about?
LAUGHT.	Now that you're writing movies for Fritz Lang...
BRECHT	I haven't sold anything yet—
LAUGHT.	I've had several offers recently...
BRECHT	You know, New York producers have been calling me non-stop for the past two weeks...ever since word got out that you're playing the lead.
LAUGHT.	I'm afraid I'm becoming too busy...
BRECHT	You're the main reason Orson Welles thinks this production is going to be the most important theatrical event of the twentieth century.
LAUGHT.	Welles likes to be in control, you know.
BRECHT	That's why you have to co-produce.
LAUGHT.	I think I'm going to go say hello to Fritz.
BRECHT	Oh, I wouldn't bother him.
LAUGHT.	No?
BRECHT	Why don't we grab some lunch?
LAUGHT.	I already ate. *(ELSA ENTERS smiling, with a big stogie in her mouth. She does not notice LAUGHTON.)*
ELSA	*(To BRECHT.)* Hello, darling.
LAUGHT.	'Darling'? *(ELSA notices LAUGHTON.)*
BRECHT	She, uh...she was talking to you.
LAUGHT.	I thought you were going to the lunch truck.

ELSA	I, uh...I just stopped in to see Fritz Lang.
LAUGHT.	About what?
ELSA	Work.
LAUGHT.	But why would you—
BRECHT	What else would one see Fritz Lang about?
LAUGHT.	Since when do you smoke cigars?
ELSA	I got it for you, darling. *(ELSA shoves cigar into LAUGHTON'S mouth.)*
LAUGHT.	Which movie were you talking about?
ELSA	I, uh...just wanted to see if he had any roles open.
BRECHT	Lang's always looking for actors.
LAUGHT.	Maybe I should go see him about a role. *(LAUGHTON walks towards LANG'S office.)*
BRECHT	He's extremely busy right now.
ELSA	That's why he, uh...just asked me to leave.
LAUGHT.	Oh, I'm sure he'll give me a couple of minutes.
BRECHT	Once you get on Lang's bad side, he'll never work with you again.
LAUGHT.	We're actually on quite friendly terms.
BRECHT	I don't think he's coming back today.
LAUGHT.	I thought he was in his office.
BRECHT	He, uh, just walked down the hall.
ELSA	A few seconds after me.
LAUGHT.	That's odd. I never saw him.
BRECHT	I'd be happy to recommend you, though.
LAUGHT.	Thanks.
ELSA	Well, nice seeing you, Brecht.
BRECHT	Yes. *(ELSA EXITS.)*
LAUGHT.	Cheers, old man. *(LAUGHTON EXITS. TOM ENTERS.)*
TOM	Hello, Breath.
BRECHT	What are you doing here?
TOM	I'm shooting a film.

BRECHT	What film?
TOM	A thriller...with Charles Laughton and Elsa Lanchester.
BRECHT	I never knew you acted in films. *(LAUGHTON ENTERS.)*
TOM	I hope to start doing theatre soon, too.

(**Projection**: FBI file on B. Brecht: According to MM-1, [blacked out] has had considerable contact with B. Brecht during the past several months at least.)

SCENE ELEVEN

(TOM'S house, several months later.)

(TOM looks out window with telescope, he wears earphones. LAUGHTON walks up to him. Lines within quotation marks are read from a draft of Galileo Galilei.*)*

LAUGHT.	Okay, are you ready to start? Tom... *(TOM does not respond.)* Are you ready.
TOM	Sure.
LAUGHT.	What are you looking at?
TOM	I, uh...I'm trying to look at the ocean.
LAUGHT.	Isn't Brecht's house in the way?
TOM	Maybe...maybe I oughta try a different window.
LAUGHT.	*(pause)* Well, are we going to rehearse?
TOM	Yes. *(TOM puts down telescope, earphones.)*
LAUGHT.	Let's start with scene two.
TOM	You know, this is like *deja vu.* I mean, lately I've been totally dedicated to writing. But in the back of my mind, I think I've always wanted to act in the theatre. Although I don't think I've ever verbalized that. But theatre, it...it just feels so right.
LAUGHT.	You've never even been on stage.
TOM	I was just in a movie.
LAUGHT.	You had two words, Tom.

TOM   I'm sure there's a lot I don't know yet, but—just holding a script in my hand, envisioning myself on the boards—I...I feel this vital connection with the art that seems so...so natural. Like it's something I excelled at in a previous life.

LAUGHT.   Why don't we start with this section right over here... Now you've just handed me a letter of introduction...

(TOM clears throat, hands LAUGHTON a piece of paper. Both TOM and LAUGHTON read their lines from their scripts. TOM'S acting is very self conscious.)

TOM   'Greetings, professor. I'm pleased to make your acquaintance. I'm...Lobby...Luby'...

LAUGHT.   Lobianco.

TOM   'Greetings, professor. I'm pleased to make your acquaintance. I'm Loco'...

LAUGHT.   Lobianco.

TOM   That's what I said.

LAUGHT.   You said loco.

TOM   I did not.

LAUGHT.   Don't worry about it.

TOM   I did not say loco.

LAUGHT.   *(Referring to letter.) (pause)* 'You travelled all the way here from France, although your mother resides in Sicily'...

TOM   *(TOM pronounces 'Sì', at first, as 'sigh'.)* 'Sì'.

LAUGHT.   *Sì.*

TOM   See?

LAUGHT.   'And you'd like to study science'?

TOM   *(TOM again pronounces 'Sì' as 'sigh'.)* 'Sì'.

LAUGHT.   *(Pointing to TOM's script.) Sì!*

TOM   Okay.

LAUGHT.   It's simple.

TOM   I know—

LAUGHT.   It's only two letters. S-i. *Sì. Sì.*

TOM	Well, I never studied German, okay?
LAUGHT.	'I can be your personal tutor...for ten scudi per week'.
TOM	'When I was in Paris, I saw a tool just like yours'.
LAUGHT.	What 'tool' are you talking about?
TOM	One like yours.
LAUGHT.	Yes, but what do you think of the tool?
TOM	Oh, I think it's quite functional... *(TOM laughs.)*
LAUGHT.	You don't understand it.
TOM	'Angela exits'.
LAUGHT.	Why did you say that?
TOM	Oh, is that *your* line?
LAUGHT.	Why would your character say that?
TOM	Because he wants Galileo to know that Angela left.
LAUGHT.	It's a stage direction.
TOM	Oh... 'I almost purchased the tool in Paris. It was a foot long'. A foot long? *(TOM smiles.)*
LAUGHT.	Just read the lines, please... 'So I assume you had a good look at this tool'. *(LAUGHTON shows TOM a sketch.)* 'Do you see any...resemblance'?
TOM	'Well, sort of. But I hadn't ever seen them prior to their appearance on the plaza just before I decided to travel to Venice'.
LAUGHT.	Let's move on to scene four. 'Esteemed lords, cardinals...this humble scholar of science has always been honored to serve you by developing scientific knowledge that has reaped great profit and prestige for the State. It thus gives me great pleasure to unveil a new invention of mine, developed in accordance with the teachings of the Bible and the Vatican... *(TOM falls asleep, eventually snores.)* Which I have named the telescope'... Tom!
TOM	Oh.
LAUGHT.	You have to stay focused.
TOM	I was just thinking about your, uh, tool...and I fell asleep.

LAUGHT.	I would hope that that wouldn't happen in the theatre.
TOM	Only if I were in the audience.
LAUGHT.	Let's jump ahead... *(Points to line near end of scene four.)* I'll read your cues.
TOM	Who's Livia?
LAUGHT	My daughter.
TOM	You have a daughter?
LAUGHT.	Galileo has a daughter... *(As a teenage girl.)* 'Father, Lobianco is eager to speak with you'.
TOM	'Your tool is a wonderful accomplishment, sir'.
LAUGHT.	*(As teenage girl.)*. 'Everyone says father's a genius'.
TOM	'He seems to be'.
LAUGHT.	*(As teenage girl.)* 'Don't you think father's tool is amazing'?
TOM	'It's an amazing *pink*'. *(TOM smiles.)* You wrote that, didn't you? *(TOM glances at LAUGHTON'S crotch.)*
LAUGHT.	Brecht and I still have to do some polishing.
TOM	You know, this is the sort of part that...that I can really sink my teeth into.
LAUGHT.	We still need to do a lot of work.
TOM	Well, you and Breath do what you have to do with the script, but I can't wait to get up there on the boards.
LAUGHT.	We have to work on your presentation.
TOM	*(Defensive.)* What's wrong with my presentation?
LAUGHT.	Nothing that can't be improved.
TOM	You don't think I can act?
LAUGHT.	No, no... I'm sure you can act. It's just that, well...you haven't done it before.
TOM	Galileo's an atheist, isn't he?
LAUGHT.	No. But his work is being suppressed by the Church, which is also running the state.
TOM	What's wrong with that?
LAUGHT.	That's exactly the sort of question Brecht wants the spectator to think about.
TOM	So the play's subversive.

LAUGHT.   It's a play. So it's much more complicated than any social statements.

TOM   I don't want to do it.

LAUGHT.   I thought you wanted to work with me.

TOM   I'd rather just concentrate on my writing.

LAUGHT.   Tom, if you play Lobianco, you're going to make connections. Chaplin's already expressed an interest in the play. Peter Lorre, who's a personal friend of Brecht's, might be playing the Pope. And it looks as if Orson Welles is going to be directing.

TOM   What's it going to pay?

LAUGHT.   Well, we'll be opening in Los Angeles. And as long as everything goes well, which it will, you'll be receiving a substantial wage once we hit Broadway.

TOM   I don't work for free.

LAUGHT.   You're not going to.

TOM   I mean, if they expect me to take time away from my writing, then I have to get—

LAUGHT.   You're not going to work for nothing. I'll make sure of it.

TOM   Is the Broadway production definite?

LAUGHT.   Just about.

TOM   So it isn't.

LAUGHT.   No, it is... We're just waiting on a couple of contracts.

TOM   Can I get you a glass of Scotch?

LAUGHT.   Yes... As long as we get right back to work... *(TOM gets two drinks.)* How do you support yourself?

TOM   Well, I, uh... I'm a writer, primarily.

LAUGHT.   What do you do for money?

TOM   I work at Hollywood Bowl... I'm in charge of the ushers.

LAUGHT.   And you're able to pay for a house in Santa Monica with that?

TOM   Well, I, uh...I have a trust fund.

LAUGHT.   We better get back to the play.

TOM   We can do it later.

LAUGHT.	You need to practice for the audition.
TOM	You're the producer, Charles.
LAUGHT.	I'm one of the producers.
TOM	I'd hate to see anything get in the way of our relationship.
LAUGHT.	Brecht doesn't give a damn about relationships.
TOM	Well, certainly you have some leverage...
LAUGHT.	You still have to be adequate during the audition on Saturday.
TOM	You don't think I'm adequate?
LAUGHT.	Tom, look, no matter what sort of leverage I try to apply, Brecht will not compromise his art.
TOM	*(pause)* You wouldn't work with a Communist, would you?
LAUGHT.	What?
TOM	Oh...I just heard something...
LAUGHT.	About Brecht?
TOM	It's probably just a rumor.
LAUGHT.	Then why don't we leave it at that and get back to rehearsing?
TOM	I'd like to, but I...I'm just too tired right now... But I have something that I've been wanting to give you. *(TOM pulls out a small box of photographs.)* It's just a little gift.
LAUGHT.	Oh.
TOM	Go ahead...open it. *(LAUGHTON opens box, looks at pictures.)*
LAUGHT.	Oh, a picture of you in a bathing suit.
TOM	Do you like it?
LAUGHT.	You look so buff.
TOM	There's more.
LAUGHT.	A picture of both of us in bathing suits...
TOM	Look at the next one.
LAUGHT.	I don't remember anyone taking this picture.
TOM	Isn't it hot?
LAUGHT.	Who took this?

TOM	Don't you remember? I had the camera set up on a tripod.
LAUGHT.	It's always on a tripod. But I've never seen anybody using it.
TOM	I was using a remote control.
LAUGHT.	You never told me you were taking photographs.
TOM	Of course I didn't tell you. That's why the pictures look so natural.
	(LAUGHTON thumbs through more pictures.)
LAUGHT.	Too natural...
TOM	Don't you like them?
LAUGHT.	Well, yes, but...I don't think I could take these home... Maybe I should just keep them here.
TOM	They're for you.
LAUGHT.	But if I take them with me, then you won't have any.
TOM	I made copies. And I have lots of other pictures of us, too. *(pause)* Let me go get 'em. *(TOM EXITS. LAUGHTON follows him.)*

(**Projection**: J. Edgar Hoover: Communists and Fascists are materialistic, totalitarian, anti-religious, degrading and inhuman. They differ little except in name. Communism has bred Fascism. Fascism spawns Communism.)

SCENE TWELVE

(BRECHT'S home.)

BRECHT	You could work with Tom for five years, twenty-four hours a day, and he still wouldn't get it.
LAUGHT.	I think we should give him another shot.
BRECHT	He'll ruin the goddamn play.
LAUGHT.	I've seen worse, even on—
BRECHT	I don't even want to discuss this anymore.
LAUGHT.	My agent thinks I should get a firm commitment on the New York performance dates.
BRECHT	*I* want a firm commitment. Welles wants to push the shows back again.

LAUGHT.   Elsa was talking to another producer who might be interested.

BRECHT   Who?

LAUGHT.   Mike Tolland.

BRECHT   Have him give me a call.

LAUGHT.   Frank Capra wants me to do a film with him in the fall.

BRECHT   What's it called?

LAUGHT.   *It's a Wonderful Life.* He wants me to play the lead.

BRECHT   With a title like *It's a Wonderful Life*, I'd be surprised if it plays for more than a couple of weeks.

LAUGHT.   At least it would pay a decent wage.

BRECHT   But then you'll be doing another hack film, and then another, and another.

LAUGHT.   If I'm going to do a play, it's crucial that I'm performing with actors with whom I want to work.

BRECHT   Make some recommendations.

LAUGHT.   Well...as far the the role of Andrea goes, I think that if you give Tom another opportunity he'll show you—

BRECHT   Tom is not going to be in *Galileo.*

(**Projection**: FBI file on B. Brecht: Los Angeles Field Office will attempt to prepare enough clear-cut evidence to determine whether...the United States Attorney...will authorize the arrest of Subject with a view to his internment or deportation. Approval granted to install technical surveillance on subject...provided full security assured.)

SCENE THIRTEEN

(TOM'S house.)

TOM   My shoulders feel awfully tight. *(LAUGHTON begins massaging TOM.)*

LAUGHT.   I still don't understand why Capra reneged on his offer.

TOM   Can you get around the neck... And the shoulder blades...

LAUGHT.   I'll tell Brecht again how right you'll be for the part.

TOM   A little lower, Charles... Oh...that feels good...

LAUGHT.   I...I don't know what else I can do.

TOM   You know, we still have to be cautious of enemy aliens.

LAUGHT.   The war's virtually over.

TOM   It's just beginning... America's major threat, now, is the enemy within. Which is a bigger challenge, actually, than World War II...

LAUGHT.   I think that's all being exaggerated.

TOM   *(LAUGHTON continues the massage.)* You know, a lot of writers and actors are being closely scrutinized right now...

LAUGHT.   It's not the most conducive environment for creating art, is it?

TOM   And with all the buzz about *Galileo Galilei*, everyone knows, now, that you've been working with Brecht.

LAUGHT.   Well, Brecht's certainly not a Soviet operative.

TOM   Do you have any evidence to support that?

LAUGHT.   We've been working together for months.

TOM   Do you know much about his work with radical exile organizations, like the Free German movement?

LAUGHT.   I haven't the foggiest...

TOM   Has he published any plays or essays critical of communism?

LAUGHT.   I never said he was critical of communism.

TOM   Perhaps you should tell someone.

LAUGHT.   What?

TOM   That Brecht isn't anti-Communist.

LAUGHT.   For what?

TOM   Either he's with us or against us.

LAUGHT.   I'm not going to compromise our relationship.

TOM   I assume that you're talking about *our* relationship, Charles. Because I'd hate to see everything come to an end because the government ends up revoking your visa.

LAUGHT.   If worse came to worse, I suppose I could always work over in England.

TOM	Once English journalists find out about a star's unusual sexual inclinations, they'll plaster it all over the newspapers. *(LAUGHTON stops massaging TOM.)*
LAUGHT.	Why would they find that out?
TOM	I don't know. But they could.
LAUGHT.	Well, I'm not going to have to work in England.
TOM	American newspapers would do the same thing. With articles, photographs.
LAUGHT.	I'm not going to betray Brecht.
TOM	As long as your work on *Galileo* is enabling you to gather information, no one's going to tamper with the play. Otherwise, I'm afraid it might be shut down.
LAUGHT.	So this is what you want to see happen?
TOM	I have nothing to do with it.
LAUGHT.	You certainly seem to know a lot.
TOM	Someone came to visit me... Because I'm Brecht's next door neighbor. And I don't want to see you get hurt.
LAUGHT.	I can't just back out of the play at this point.
TOM	You'll be fine, Charles...as long as you provide information about any of Brecht's activities that might seem anti-American.
LAUGHT.	I'd probably forget most of what he says.
TOM	It doesn't matter. They'll have you wear a wire.
LAUGHT.	A wire?
TOM	Or maybe they'll have you hold one... Microphones are so small these days, they can stick them in almost anything, like...like a cigar.
LAUGHT.	For all I know, the production's not even going to happen.
TOM	It has to happen. Because it's going to enable you to get the information on Brecht that you've been witholding.
LAUGHT.	I haven't witheld anything.
TOM	You don't want to be blacklisted...
LAUGHT.	Well, no, of course not. But I'm not about to spy on a friend.
TOM	You don't have any choice at this point.

SCENE FOURTEEN

(BRECHT'S front yard.)

(**Projection**: The new, American atomic bomb destroyed the entire Japanese city of Hiroshima in a single blast....350,000 innocent people are there one moment...and wiped out the next.)

(ANGEL ENTERS, working.)

ANGEL   I thought you might like some more of these. *(ANGEL gives BRECHT a bunch of cigars.)*

BRECHT   Wonderful... At least let me give you a dollar.

ANGEL   No.

BRECHT   You've got kids to support.

ANGEL   The spirits won't accept money.

BRECHT   *(BRECHT chuckles.)* It's just tobacco.

ANGEL   *(With great purpose.).* It's *not* just tobacco... And while it's burning I want you to focus on the cigar's smoke, the tobacco's spirit.

BRECHT   All I ever think about is where to put the ashes.

ANGEL   *(ANGEL says the following lines with powerful, prophetic conviction.)* Then you have to pay closer attention. To the moment. While everything's burning, in flux. If you see only the ash, you can't understand the present. If you see nothing but fire, you'll never grasp the past. But the connection between fire and ash, past and present, becomes visible—at times—in the smoke, as a constellation. But you have to seize the image the second it flits by or it's going to disappear.

BRECHT   You sure there's only tobacco in these? *(BRECHT writes, ANGEL finishes doing yardwork, EXITS. Eventually, LAUGHTON ENTERS, with his raincoat's collar pulled up around his face. He's carrying several newspapers, a huge cigar that contains a microphone. LAUGHTON handles the cigar awkwardly, at times.)* Laughton.

LAUGHT.   Don't say my name so loudly.

BRECHT   It's not supposed to rain today, is it?

LAUGHT.   I...I don't want anyone to recognize me...

BRECHT   What's the matter?

LAUGHT.   Did you see this? *(LAUGHTON points to one of his newspapers.)*

BRECHT   It's hard to believe that a civilzed person, never mind a 'democratic' government, would utilize science to murder hundreds of thousands of people.

LAUGHT.   Well, there's that, too... But there's also something about me in here... It's in all the papers. *(LAUGHTON hands BRECHT papers. BRECHT reads.)* The *L.A. Times, Variety...* Right on the front page... *(BRECHT reads.)* I lost a ten by fifteen foot section of my property. Gone, caput, right down the side of the cliff...

BRECHT   Some things you can't control.

LAUGHT.   You see what they're saying in those articles? I just want to crawl under a rock and die.

BRECHT   *(BRECHT reads the words within quotation marks.)* 'The actor Charles Laughton recently lost a portion of his garden in Pacific Palisades during a slight landslide'. So what?

LAUGHT.   Look at the gossip columns. *(BRECHT looks at a gossip column.)* They're equating the crumbling of my garden with the faltering of my career.

BRECHT   *(pause)* It doesn't say that here.

LAUGHT.   Read between the lines... Industry people are looking at the papers right now and laughing... Because those articles are just reinforcing what studio execs have been thinking about me... And this is only the beginning... There's a subterranean stream undermining everything. So the world, my career is going to continue to fall apart, right beneath my feet... I'm just so ashamed right now... Oh, I...I'm sorry. I shouldn't be troubling you with all this...

BRECHT   You're over-reacting, Laughton. You're an accomplished actor...

LAUGHT.   All I've been getting lately are offers to play supporting roles, for people like Marjorie Main and Wallace Beery...

BRECHT   That's going to change once people see you in the play.

LAUGHT.   There's still the subterranean stream.

BRECHT   The L.A. run of *Galileo's* already sold out—for three weeks—because of you.

LAUGHT.   But it's not going to make it to Broadway now.

BRECHT   I just talked to Mike Tolland yesterday.

LAUGHT.   He called you?

BRECHT   Broadway's a done deal.

LAUGHT.   You talked to Tolland before the bomb was dropped, right?

BRECHT   What difference does it make?

LAUGHT.   Nobody's going to produce a controversial play about science right after the world's worst scientific atrocity.

BRECHT   All we have to do is help the audience to see the parallels between the dawn of science and the birth of the atomic bomb.

LAUGHT.   Galileo's discovery didn't kill hundreds of thousands of people.

BRECHT   In both cases, scientists let themselves be manipulated at the expense of—

LAUGHT.   Galileo wasn't manipulated.

BRECHT   He caved in to the Church.

LAUGHT.   One has to bend a bit sometimes.

BRECHT   Galileo's a coward, just like Oppenheimer.

LAUGHT.   Well, I'm not about to play him as a cowering wretch. *(BRECHT takes out a lighter.)*

BRECHT   Let me give you a light.

LAUGHT.   *(LAUGHTON pulls his cigar back.)* No.

BRECHT   What good's a cigar if you don't light it?

LAUGHT.   I...I just feel like holding it...to calm my nerves.

BRECHT   I want you to try out some new lines. *(BRECHT hands LAUGHTON an altered monologue.)*

LAUGHT.   *(LAUGHTON looks a monologue.)* I thought this speech was pretty well set...

BRECHT   I had to make a few changes. *(BRECHT points to a passage.)* Why don't you start right here?

LAUGHT. *(LAUGHTON reads, performs.)* 'Allowing force, or those in power, to affect one's research can alter science irretrievably, and the latest discoveries may merely create new discord. Progress that fails to benefit the whole will always pit science not with but against the majority. Thus, earnest applause for the latest discovery will soon be eclipsed by the relentless clamor of unprecedented global suffering'.

BRECHT Good.

LAUGHT. This 'global suffering'...it refers to the atomic bomb...

BRECHT That's what the play's about now.

LAUGHT. The way you discuss scientific progress, the ways that machines and science don't really help, but exploit... It's...it's... *(LAUGHTON becomes mute.)*

BRECHT What? *(LAUGHTON gives thumbs up sign.)* You like it? *(LAUGHTON nods yes.)* So you like the change?

LAUGHT. *(LAUGHTON talks into cigar.)* Well, no.

BRECHT You don't think it works? *(LAUGHTON nods yes.)* You do?

LAUGHT. *(LAUGHTON talks into cigar.)* No.

BRECHT But you just nodded your head that it does.

LAUGHT. No I didn't.

BRECHT You feeling okay?

LAUGHT. *(LAUGHTON feigns laryngitis.)* I...I'm coming down with laryngitis... So I'm trying not to talk too much.

BRECHT Would you like some water?

LAUGHT. Do you have anything stronger?

BRECHT Scotch?

LAUGHT. Well, I really shouldn't...but if you insist... *(BRECHT EXITS, TOM appears from behind a bush.)*

TOM Hello, Charles.

LAUGHT. What are you doing here?

TOM I, uh...I'm looking for a golf ball.

LAUGHT. I didn't know you played golf.

TOM   You need to ask more pointed questions.

LAUGHT.   I really don't want to participate in this.

TOM   That was just recorded.

LAUGHT.   *(LAUGHTON looks at cigar.)* Shit. I keep forgetting.

TOM   Think of your career. *(TOM begins to EXIT.)*

LAUGHT.   Maybe I should just leave.

TOM   Get some more information first. *(BRECHT ENTERS with Scotch.)*

BRECHT   Tom... You're not still looking for a part in the play, are you?

TOM   I, uh... I was just looking for a golf ball. *(TOM EXITS. BRECHT hands LAUGHTON a drink.)*

LAUGHT.   Thanks.

BRECHT   *Nichts zu danken. (LAUGHTON downs drink.)*

LAUGHT.   I'm sorry, but I'm going to have to call it a day. *(LAUGHTON begins to EXIT.)*

BRECHT   Make sure you get some rest.

LAUGHT.   *(LAUGHTON stops. During rest of scene, his 'laryngitis' comes and goes.)* Oh, ummm...I've been meaning to ask you... *(LAUGHTON is handling his cigar in an awkward manner as he tries to use it to record BRECHT'S words.)* What does the play have to do with the Free German movement?

BRECHT   Nothing... Why?

LAUGHT.   Oh, I was just wondering...

BRECHT   Right now the Free German movement's main concern is that no one associated with Hitler has any power during reconstruction.

LAUGHT.   What about the Communists?

BRECHT   Well, Germany would certainly be better off with the Communists in power than the Fascists, wouldn't it?

LAUGHT.   I don't know.

BRECHT   Well, that's what you've said before.

LAUGHT.   I never said that.

BRECHT   You said it last week.

LAUGHT.   You must be mistaken.

BRECHT	I'm *not* mistaken.
LAUGHT.	*(LAUGHTON speaks into cigar.)* Germany needs, uh, American democracy.
BRECHT	If they only look to the US for help, then all they're going to get is imperialism, right?
LAUGHT.	I...I don't think so.
BRECHT	Why are you changing your stance all of a sudden?
LAUGHT.	I've always felt this way.
BRECHT	Is your voice coming back?
LAUGHT.	*(LAUGHTON feigns oncoming laryngitis again.)* No, no, not at all...
BRECHT	I've never seen anyone hold a cigar like that.
LAUGHT.	Well, I...I guess it's...it's a bit awkward for me...because it's larger than what I'm used to.
BRECHT	*(BRECHT holds up a light, LAUGHTON pulls cigar away.)* Why are you bothering with the thing if you're not going to smoke it?
LAUGHT.	I...I need something to occupy my hands. And smoking's not good for my laryngitis. *(LAUGHTON'S 'laryngitis' becomes worse.)*
BRECHT	You haven't had any vocal problems at rehearsal...
LAUGHT.	Not with my voice... But, to be honest, rehearsing has become so stressful lately...because you're so insistent on having me deliver the monologues in a manner that's inconsistent with my interpretation of what you've written.
BRECHT	If you had a better grasp of Galileo's faint-heartedness, you'd be able—
LAUGHT.	I cannot perform Galileo that way.
BRECHT	You have to.
LAUGHT.	I can't.
BRECHT	If you just took my direction...
LAUGHT.	*(Definitively.)* I'm not going to do it.
BRECHT	What?
LAUGHT.	I quit.
BRECHT	You can't quit.
LAUGHT.	There are plenty of other actors...

BRECHT	We've been working on this for nearly a year.
LAUGHT.	I refuse to make the character something it's not.
BRECHT	We can talk about this.
LAUGHT.	You never listen.
BRECHT	Why don't we get together tomorrow morning?
LAUGHT.	For what?
BRECHT	We can work this out, Laughton.
LAUGHT.	You have to trust my instincts.
BRECHT	We can meet at your house.
LAUGHT.	Oh...I'd prefer to come here.
BRECHT	Your place is so much more pleasant.
LAUGHT.	Not since the landslide took my big trees... I mean, I just dread going back into my house now, especially during the day... It...it feels so different since the old oak went. There's so much light. Everywhere. It's as if the whole place has changed... This morning, the sun was pouring in through the windows, brightening corners that have never seen the light of day... It's...it's really unbearable for me.
BRECHT	We'll pull down the shades. *(BRECHT pats LAUGHTON on the back. LAUGHTON EXITS. BRECHT writes for a while. Eventually, ELSA ENTERS.)*

(**Projection**: FBI file on B. Brecht: FBI recommends Brecht's internment to Assistant Attorney General Attilio di Girolamo....This action should be taken without delay.)

ELSA	Brecht, darling.
BRECHT	You never told me you were coming over.
ELSA	Do I need an invitation now?
BRECHT	Well...there's the children...
ELSA	I brought them each a little gift.
BRECHT	They're not home at the moment.
ELSA	Oh, no?
BRECHT	They went to the store with my wife.

ELSA	I'm so excited about *Mother Courage*. I'm ready to dive right into it.
BRECHT	We have to get *Galileo* up first.
ELSA	We can work together in the evening, after rehearsals.
BRECHT	I wouldn't want Charles to get jealous.
ELSA	I've decided to leave Charles.
BRECHT	What?
ELSA	I have to.
BRECHT	I thought you and Charles had an understanding.
ELSA	We do. But he's never home anymore, anyway. And he seems to be encouraging me to leave. *(ELSA runs her hands through BRECHT'S hair.)* You don't mind, do you? Now I'll have more time to spend with you.
BRECHT	I don't know...
ELSA	Why don't we go inside for a while?
BRECHT	Ruth Berlau just called. She's on her way back to California.
ELSA	I hope you told her that you're already spoken for.
BRECHT	*(pause)* I couldn't.
ELSA	What!?
BRECHT	I've known her for nearly ten years. And then there's my wife, the children... And you, of course. Which is why I discouraged her from returning... But I can handle only so many things at one time...
ELSA	As soon as something else comes along, you want to drop me like a hot potato...
BRECHT	I didn't expect Berlau to come back to Los Angeles.
ELSA	It's not as if you're married... Well, not to Berlau anyway.
BRECHT	You just have to be patient...till all the dust settles... And I have to be going now.
ELSA	You're just walking away...
BRECHT	I'm not walking—
ELSA	After all I went through for you.
BRECHT	We were just fucking.
ELSA	Who do you think secured you a producer for *Galileo*?

BRECHT	Laughton found him.
ELSA	No, it was me... When I heard you were having trouble with Welles, I went to visit Mike Tolland and I convinced him to produce your play.
BRECHT	*Galileo Galilei's* going to be on Broadway—and it's even becoming a movie now—because of the writing.
ELSA	The writing? *(ELSA laughs.)* Tolland hasn't even read it.
BRECHT	Bullshit.
ELSA	I've been telling him that he didn't have to. Because I know that he hates being associated with anything 'controversial'. Especially with Congress working so dilligently to ferret out 'reds' in Hollywood.
BRECHT	Berlau's going to be back in New York soon.
ELSA	I think I'm going to encourage Tolland to read your play. *(ELSA EXITS.)*

(**Projection**: FBI file on R. Berlau: Agent Hood requests blanket authorization for the installation of a microphone surveillance in whichever unit of Chalet Motor Inn Berlau might reside after relocating from the Beverly Hills home of P. Lorre.)

SCENE FIFTEEN

(Chalet Motor Inn.)

(BERLAU is very pregnant; she's sweating. Nearby is a new Leica camera.)

BERLAU	*(Upset.)* I feel like a pregnant nun who's been sequestered, so as not to bring shame to the order—
BRECHT	Now don't get upset again.
BERLAU	For the past six weeks you forced me to live with a morphine addict...while people kept wandering in and out of the house all night...sitting out by the pool drinking, smoking...
BRECHT	Everything's going to work out.
BERLAU	How? Are you going to keep me and the baby locked up in this fleabag hotel until he's twenty-one years old?

BRECHT   At least you're close by now.

BERLAU   Your gutter's even closer by. Is that where you want me to move next?

BRECHT   Look, with Broadway up in the air right now, and Laughton...I'm doing the best I can.

BERLAU   For the first time since we met, I'm about to produce something that's indisputably mine. And you keep trying to cover it up.

BRECHT   It's going to be different once the baby arrives.

BERLAU   If you don't get me out of this hell-hole by next Friday, I swear to God I'm going to call all of your friends and tell them how hard you've been working to make sure nobody knows that I've been carrying your child for eight months.

BRECHT   You're getting an apartment.

BERLAU   By next week.

BRECHT   *(pause)* Let me finish showing you the manuscripts I want you to photograph.

BERLAU   I don't feel like doing this right now.

BRECHT   It'll take five minutes.

BERLAU   I'm exhausted.

BRECHT   If I can finish showing you tonight, you won't have to think about it again. Till after the baby.

BERLAU   What do you want to name it?

BRECHT   *(pause)* Whatever you want.

BERLAU   If it's a boy I'm going to name him Michel. After the baby in *The Caucasian Chalk Circle*.

BRECHT   All my plays from the twenties are in this box over here. Which is where I want you to start.

BERLAU   It's so hot in here.

BRECHT   Hot?

BERLAU   You know, there's an ice-cream parlor right down the block. We can sit right out on the sidewalk.

BRECHT   We're in the middle of Santa Monica.

BERLAU   I *have to* get out of this room.

BRECHT	I just want to show you—
BERLAU	Now!
BRECHT	Let's...let's go sit by the pool.
BERLAU	I want to go have some ice cream.
BRECHT	I'll go out and get it.
BERLAU	I don't want to sit here all by myself.
BRECHT	I'll be back in a minute.
BERLAU	I need to be around people.
BRECHT	It's just another month.
BERLAU	*(Agitated.)* I have to go out and get some ice cream.
BRECHT	Ruth, relax.
BERLAU	Right now!
BRECHT	I can go out and get it.
BERLAU	*(Desperate.)* Take me out of this room, goddamn it!
BRECHT	Okay, okay... Where's your coat?
BERLAU	Coat? It's a hundred degrees outside.
BRECHT	I just thought you'd want to cover yourself up.
BERLAU	I'm not covering anything.
BRECHT	*(pause)* Okay...
BERLAU	The baby cannot remain couped up in squalid rooms, hidden beneath overcoats. *(Phone rings.)* It needs fresh air.
BRECHT	*(BRECHT picks up phone.)* Hello... Laughton...Laughton...
BERLAU	Ohhh...
BRECHT	Disconnected, damn it. *(BRECHT hangs up phone.)*
BERLAU	Ahhh...
BRECHT	What's the matter?
BERLAU	I...I just have a little indigestion.
BRECHT	Why don't we take the car?
BERLAU	I want to walk.
BRECHT	C'mon. *(BERLAU suddenly writhes in response to sudden stomach pain.)*

BERLAU	Aaahhh...
BRECHT	Ruth...
BERLAU	Ohhh... Aaaahhh...
BRECHT	Sit down. *(BRECHT helps her sit.)*
BERLAU	Aaaaahhhhh.... Uhhhhhhh...
BRECHT	You're going to be okay.
BERLAU	Ooooohhhhh...
BRECHT	Did...did your water break?
BERLAU	Aaaahhhh.... Ohhh... *(BERLAU checks to see if her water broke.)* No...no water... Ohhh...ohhh...
BRECHT	What's the matter?
BERLAU	I... I don't know. Aaaaaahhhhhh.... Aaahhh... Ohhhhhh...
BRECHT	C'mon, I'll...I'll take you to the hospital. *(BRECHT tries to help her up, to no avail.)*
BERLAU	Oh, no... Aaahhh... It hurts too much... Aaahhh...
BRECHT	I...I can try to carry you. *(BRECHT tries to carry her.)*
BERLAU	Ohhh... Aaaahhh... No, no... Ohhhhhh... *(Phone rings. BERLAU continues reacting to pain, which gradually increases.)*
BRECHT	Hello... Laughton...
BERLAU	Aaahhhhhh...
BRECHT	What? Tolland's backing out of *Galileo* because he doesn't like the script...
BERLAU	Ohhhhhh... Aaahhh...
BRECHT	No, you can't do a movie. We'll get another producer...
BERLAU	Aaahhhhhhhhh... Ohhh...
BRECHT	She's all right...she...she just has a bit of indigestion...
BERLAU	Aaahhhhhhhhhhhhhh...
BRECHT	I'll talk to you later. *(BRECHT hangs up phone.)*
BERLAU	Aaahhh. I...I feel like I'm going to burst. Ohhhhhh... Ohhhhhh... Ah. Ohhhhhhhhhhhh... Ahhhhhhhhh...
BRECHT	I'll...I'll call the doctor.

BERLAU	Call an ambulance. Aaahhh...
BRECHT	Okay, okay.
BERLAU	Ohhhhhhhhhhhhhhhhhhhhhhhhhhhhhhhh... Aaahhhhhhhh...
BRECHT	Where the hell's the phone book?
BERLAU	Call the operator.
BRECHT	*(BRECHT picks up phone.)* Hello...operator... Tom?
BERLAU	Aaahhhhhhhhhhhhhhhhhhhhhh...
BRECHT	What are you doing on this line?
BERLAU	Call the ambulance!!! *(BRECHT hangs up phone.)*
BRECHT	Okay!
BERLAU	Aaaaaaaaaaaaaaaaaahhhhhhhhhhhhhhhh....
BRECHT	Hello, operator. There's a pregnant woman here who needs an ambulance.
BERLAU	Ohhhhhhhhh...
BRECHT	Chalet Motor Inn, 3220 Wilshire.
BERLAU	Aaahhhhhh...
BRECHT	No, I am not her husband.
BERLAU	Aaahhhhhh...
BRECHT	Just hurry up, please!
BERLAU	Ohhhhhhhhhh... Aaahhhhhhhhhhhh...
BRECHT	You're going to be okay, Ruth.
BERLAU	Aaaaaahhhhhhhhh... Ohhhhhh... *(BLACKOUT.)*

(**Projection**: FBl file on R. Berlau: Hotel room contained boxes of Brecht's manuscripts. Contents of Berlau's suitcase included various supplies of photographic papers, 35mm film, assorted infant attire, 0-6 months.)

SCENE SIXTEEN

(LANG'S office.)

BRECHT	There's a revolutionary cigar roller forced to mow lawns...for low pay...like thousands of other Hispanics. But then he organizes the yardworkers...

LANG	Brecht.
BRECHT	And they all go out on strike.
LANG	Brecht! The people who green-light movies like having their lawns cut every week. Cheaply. *(LANG begins to EXIT.)*
BRECHT	I have several more scenarios—
LANG	I don't want to hear them.
BRECHT	Please, Lang, just give me five minutes.
LANG	It's unneccessary. *(LANG looks at his watch.)*
BRECHT	Look, I'm sorry I was late, but I couldn't help it. I had to stop at the hospital.
LANG	For what?
BRECHT	I...I had to drop off a friend of mine.
LANG	Anything serious?
BRECHT	No, no, not at all. And I think I deserve a few more minutes to discuss my new movie idea—
LANG	Brecht, relax. I've been shopping around your Heydrich the Hangman scenario. The movie's going to be called *Hangmen Also Hang*.
BRECHT	That's unacceptable.
LANG	It's already been decided.
BRECHT	It's my movie.
LANG	No...it's your idea. And once your idea's sold, it belongs to whomever paid for it.
BRECHT	I haven't sold it yet.
LANG	You're about to sell it.
BRECHT	Then it has to be under my terms.
LANG	*(LANG smiles.)* Brecht...you haven't even written anything yet.
BRECHT	When do I get paid?
LANG	You'll get half the money up front. Five thousand. But you have to write a treatment first. And we have to finish this thing before people lose interest in war.
BRECHT	The war's over.

LANG   Brecht, the war is never over. Just the faces change. But you'll have to make the story a bit more light-hearted.

BRECHT   The movie's about Nazis.

LANG   I know. And we can keep much of your story. But Edgar Bergen's under contract here... So one of the anti-Fascists is going to be played by Charlie McCarthy. *(Looks at watch.)* And I'm running late for, I don't know...something. *(LANG EXITS.)*

(**Projection**: FBI file on B. Brecht: Brecht's treatment for the film *Hangmen Also Die* shows a familiarity through personal experience with all the tricks of an underground movement: never tell the police anything, establish alibis so as to fool the police, work very secretly, guard against informers. **Internment of subject imminent, upon Justice Department approval**.)

SCENE SEVENTEEN

(BERLAU'S apartment.)

(BERLAU is taking pictures of manuscript pages. BRECHT reads the paper, smokes a cigar.)

BERLAU   Just a few more plays to go...

BRECHT   And then we can start on the journals...

BERLAU   You want the journals, as well?

BRECHT   Everything must be preserved.

BERLAU   Then I guess I'll move on to the journals for a while... *(BERLAU takes out journals, eventually starts photographing them.)*

BRECHT   Just try to keep it all in order. *(BRECHT jots down some notes now and then. BERLAU'S work pace continues to increase as she photographs journal pages.)*

BERLAU   The air in here is so stifling.

BRECHT   I'll open the windows.

BERLAU   They're painted shut.

BRECHT   I'll have to pick you up a fan at Woolworth's. (pause) This place isn't so bad. You have your own kitchen here, a darkroom for developing photographs...

BERLAU	I can't wait to start taking pictures of people for a change.
BRECHT	We'll get pictures of every rehearsal, the shows—of every one of my plays, eventually. *(BERLAU continues taking pictures. Eventually, a journal passage catches her attention.)*
BERLAU	What's this journal entry about?
BRECHT	If you're going to start reading everything now, you're never going to finish.
BERLAU	*(Reading.)* 'sept. 4th. surgeon operates on ruth. the bill: forty-five dollars'.
BRECHT	A lot of that writing, I'm not even thinking.
BERLAU	You're always thinking.
BRECHT	That's...that's just a mindless notation.
BERLAU	I was in the hospital then.
BRECHT	They're just notes.
BERLAU	You paid absolutely nothing towards the doctors' bills.
BRECHT	You know I didn't have any—
BERLAU	If it were up to the doctors I'd be resting in the hospital right now...
BRECHT	Ruth, you've been doing fine.
BERLAU	You make it sound as if I had just had a corn removed...
BRECHT	What happened, Ruth, it—
BERLAU	What's the forty-five dollars for?
BRECHT	Well...the funeral home, they—
BERLAU	We never had a funeral.
BRECHT	*(pause)* He was two days old.
BERLAU	And nobody even knows he was born.
BRECHT	We'll adopt a child once we get back to Europe.
BERLAU	Michel needs to have a funeral.
BRECHT	It will just make things worse.
BERLAU	I want him to have a funeral, damn it... In a Catholic Church...with altar boys...flowers.
BRECHT	Ruth, right now, you...you just need to take it easy.

BERLAU   When? After I'm done photographing another two thousand pages? *(BERLAU works.)* I cannot continue to hide everything. *You* can't.

BRECHT   Once we're in Germany, we're not going to hide—

BERLAU   What did you spend the forty-five dollars on?

BRECHT   *(pause)* Michel's cremation.

BERLAU   *(pause) (Softly.)* Cremation... *(pause)* You couldn't pay for doctors' visits, my train ticket, a decent place for me to stay— *(BERLAU take pictures of manuscript pages at a furious pace.)*

BRECHT   Maybe I don't deal with death well, all right—

BERLAU   Or *life.*

BRECHT   I...I never acknowledged the death of another son, either.

BERLAU   What?

BRECHT   Apparently, while my son Frank was watching a film with his infantry, the movie theatre was fire-bombed.

BERLAU   Oh, my God...

BRECHT   He was fighting on the wrong side.

BERLAU   I'm on the wrong side. *(BERLAU snaps photos of manuscript pages at an insanely rapid pace.)*

BRECHT   (pause) Ruth, relax... Ruth...

BERLAU   I'll relax when I'm dead. *(BERLAU'S work pace intensifies.)*

BRECHT   There's no need to do this now.

BERLAU   Don't you want your work to live on for eternity?

BRECHT   Well, I don't think all my writing should end up in the waste heap of history.

BERLAU   You mean like two of your sons. *(BERLAU works harder, faster.)*

BRECHT   Stop, goddamn it.

BERLAU   You couldn't take so much as one picture of our child, could you? But you want me to spend months, years, the rest of my miserable life photographing your words, actors doing exactly what you've told them—

BRECHT   Give me the camera, damn it. *(pause)* Give it to me!

BERLAU	Instead of taking pictures, maybe we should just burn everything... Shovel all the ashes into a cheap vase... *(BRECHT eventually grabs camera away from BERLAU.)*
BRECHT	You need to get some rest.
BERLAU	I want to finish.
BRECHT	Ruth...Ruth... *(BRECHT caresses BERLAU.)*
BERLAU	Don't touch me!
BRECHT	Fine. Fine! Maybe I should just stay away from here. Is that what you want?
BERLAU	*(pause)* Don't desert me...
BRECHT	I would never do that.
BERLAU	I swear I'll go mad. *(BRECHT embraces and kisses her.)* Ohhh...Bertolt.
BRECHT	*(Eventually, BRECHT begins to break away.)* I have to drop off a press release. *(BERLAU pulls him back, holds him hard.)*
BERLAU	No. *(They embrace again, kiss. Eventually, BRECHT pulls away.)*
BRECHT	I'll stop back later, okay? *(BRECHT EXITS.)*
BERLAU	I preserve all of your works, which for you is a matter of life and death. But still...again, I lead with a torch...my burning right hand, as I call into the night...'Bertolt'.

(**Projections**: FBI file on B. Brecht: Chairman of House Un-American Activities Committee, will subpoena subject to testify in Congress. Postpone FBI interview with subject and possible internment in light of his pending HUAC appearance.)

SCENE EIGHTEEN

(TOM'S house.)

(TOM is sporting a flashy, new suit.)

TOM	At least you're off the hook now.
LAUGHT.	I can't even look Brecht in the eye anymore, my career's in ruins... I've lost half of my property to a landslide...

TOM   Compared to the war that we're battling against communism, which you're helping us to win, Charles, your personal problems are piddling.

LAUGHT. I still haven't seen Brecht do anything un-American.

TOM   We'll find that out in a couple of months.

LAUGHT. I told you, I'm not doing this anymore.

TOM   You've done enough, Charles. HUAC thinks they have enough dirt on Brecht now to call him to Washington.

LAUGHT. You told me that me doing what I did wouldn't have any adverse affect on the play.

TOM   It won't. As long as Brecht can answer the questions properly.

LAUGHT. My name's on the play.

TOM   You're going to be fine, Charles. As long as you're not implicated in Brecht's testimony.

LAUGHT. Why would Brecht implicate me?

TOM   He wouldn't. Unless he knows you were spying on him.

LAUGHT. I can't believe I did this.

TOM   You did what you had to do.

LAUGHT. And now what's left?

TOM   *(pause)* Your career.

LAUGHT. This wonderful relationship...

TOM   Oh...I just accepted a government position in Washington. With the Office of Censorship. So I'm afraid our relationship's over.

SCENE NINETEEN

(Coronet Theatre. A couch sits beneath a sheet.)

(LAUGHTON rehearses a monologue. He is visibly nervous. He has his hands in his pockets and inadvertently plays with his testicles while performing his lines.)

100

LAUGHT.   *(BERLAU snaps pictures.)* 'Due to her gullibility, the peasant's struggle to support her children will never subside'. *(LAUGHTON loses his temper.)* Can you please stop making noise with that camera?

BRECHT   Relax, Laughton.

LAUGHT.   We don't even have a proper set yet.

BRECHT   It's being built.

LAUGHT.   I need to interact with Galileo's surroundings. To see Galileo's furniture, sit on it, as Galileo did. I mean, I'm sure Galileo never had a sheet draped over his couch.

BRECHT   Fine. Take it off. *(LAUGHTON pulls sheet off couch.)*

LAUGHT.   *(LAUGHTON realizes that the couch was formerly his.)* Where did you get that?

BRECHT   The Salvation Army.

BERLAU   It's perfect, isn't it?

LAUGHT.   It's...it's not right.

BRECHT   It's going to be fine.

LAUGHT.   We have to replace it. I mean, I can't—

BRECHT   Stop worrying about things that you can't control and focus on your goddamn acting. *(LAUGHTON readies himself.)*

LAUGHT.   'Intimidation encircles the scientist but he, too, must eat. What's his motivation to discover'?

BRECHT   Why are you so anxious today?

LAUGHT.   *(pause)* 'I always believed that the purpose of scientific exploration was to improve the world'.

BRECHT   Focus on the implications of the words.

LAUGHT.   How can I focus when you keep interrupting? *(LAUGHTON continues.)*

BRECHT   Proceed.

LAUGHT.   'But improvement'... *(LAUGHTON clears throat, etc.)* Do you mind if I get some water?

BRECHT   I'd like to get through the monologue. *(LAUGHTON'S pocketed hand becomes more fidgety.)*

LAUGHT.	My throat's incredibly dry right now and I'm afraid if I—
BRECHT	Go get some water, damn it! *(LAUGHTON EXITS.)* Jesus Christ... I've gotta tell him to take his hands out of his pockets.
BERLAU	Don't. He's nervous enough.
BRECHT	The audience will be laughing at him.
BERLAU	If you say anything, you're going to destroy his confidence.
BRECHT	I can't have him standing up there playing with his balls for three hours.
BERLAU	I'll tell the wardrobe girl to sew up his pockets. But don't say anything. *(BERLAU EXITS.)*
BRECHT	Goddamn sensitive actors... *(LAUGHTON ENTERS.)* Let me hear the last few lines of the final monologue.
LAUGHT.	I can't gain proper momentum unless I start from the top—
BRECHT	Just give me the last few lines...from 'During that'.
LAUGHT.	*(LAUGHTON clears throat.)* Give me a moment. *(He clears his throat again. Walks away.)*
BRECHT	*(pause)* Are you okay?
LAUGHT.	I'll...I'll be all right... *(LAUGHTON clears throat again.)* 'During the decisive moment if...if I had stood up for my principles, I could have altered the course of history. I now realize that I...I did not have to act as I did. But I capitulated to those in power'.
BRECHT	You finally seem guilty. As if you've done something completely unacceptable.
LAUGHT.	I have.
BRECHT	Your character has.
LAUGHT.	So have I.
BRECHT	It's your character, all right? Your character.
LAUGHT.	But there isn't much difference—
BRECHT	You are not your fucking character.
LAUGHT.	*(pause)* Maybe I am.
BRECHT	In epic theatre, character and actor must always remain separate.
LAUGHT.	Well, if one's in a particular situation... *(BERLAU ENTERS.)*

BRECHT	It doesn't matter. If you 'become' the character, the audience will empathize with you, as an individual, at the expense of understanding the play's political implications.
LAUGHT.	Well, I am an individual, and I—
BRECHT	I don't give a shit about individuals. I'm concerned with history, class struggle...
LAUGHT.	'I...I feel compelled, now, to divulge the truth. I sold out all that my work had stood for. Any human who chooses to act as I have...deserves to be banished from the face of the earth'. *(LAUGHTON begins to EXIT.)*
BRECHT	Laughton, it's working... You finally understand Galileo's cowardness.
ANGEL	*(ANGEL ENTERS.)* Brecht.
BRECHT	I'm in the middle of rehearsal.
ANGEL	Something very terrible has happened.
BRECHT	Who told you I was here?
ANGEL	My baby, she's ill. She's very ill, Brecht.
BRECHT	I'm sorry to hear that.
ANGEL	I...I have to get home to Cuba see my baby.
BRECHT	Do you know anyone else who can mow the lawn?
ANGEL	The doctor, he says she might not last through the weekend.
BERLAU	Oh, my god.
LAUGHT.	Jesus...
ANGEL	I need to leave for Cuba, before it's too late.
BRECHT	Well, don't let me hold you back.
ANGEL	Please, I...I need two hundred dollars for a plane ticket.
BRECHT	Well...
ANGEL	Please, Brecht.
BRECHT	I wish I could help you.
ANGEL	My baby... It's very critical...
BRECHT	If there's anything else I could do...
ANGEL	I...I just need two hundred dollars, today... *(LAUGHTON takes out cash.)*
BRECHT	I thought it wasn't safe for you to go back.

ANGEL	It doesn't matter.
BRECHT	You shouldn't be flying home right now if that's going to hinder the revolution.
ANGEL	If I can't take care of my child, or at least try—to do whatever I possibly can—then the revolution, it's...meaningless.
BRECHT	Here's a five spot. *(BRECHT gives ANGEL money.)*
ANGEL	You owe me ten for the lawn.
BRECHT	You'll have to go talk to my wife.
LAUGHT.	Here. *(LAUGHTON hands ANGEL three one-hundred-dollar bills.)*
ANGEL	Oh, thank you, sir. Thank you. *(ANGEL EXITS.)*
BRECHT	You didn't just give him two hundred dollars...
BERLAU	Three hundred. *(MARSHAL, who has had a bit to drink, ENTERS. BRECHT and BERLAU do not see him at first.)* That was so nice of you, Charles.
LAUGHT.	You don't mind if I leave now, do you?
BRECHT	No, because you finally understand your character. (LAUGHTON EXITS.)
BERLAU	Laughton's going to be fine.
MARSHAL	Uh, excuse me, sir... Are you, uh, Berth-tawlt Breeched?
BRECHT	No.
MARSHAL	You're not?
BRECHT	I'm Bertolt Brecht.
MARSHAL	That's what I meant... I, uh... Do you mind if I sit down?
BRECHT	No, not at all.
MARSHAL	I been doin' this all goddamn day... For several months... All over California...
BERLAU	Can I get you a glass of water? *(MARSHAL sniffs the air.)*
BRECHT	How about some whiskey?
MARSHAL	Whiskey sounds good.
BRECHT	*(BRECHT takes out a flask, pours whiskey.)* Here.
MARSHAL	Somethin' smells funny...
BRECHT	It's just a little musty in here.
MARSHAL	To your health. *(MARSHAL downs a shot.)*
BRECHT	Have another. *(MARSHAL takes another shot.)*

MARSHAL   I'm sorry about this, but—you understand—a man's gotta eat. And this is my

                    job... So, uh... *(MARSHAL hands papers to BRECHT, who looks them over.)*

                    Would you mind signin' right here, please?

BRECHT   What is it?

MARSHAL   A summons to appear in front of, uh... *(MARSHAL reads.)* The Honorable J.

                    Thomas Parnell... In Washington. You got to be there on, uh...October 30th...

BERLAU   Parnell's the Chairman of HUAC. *(BRECHT signs paper.)*

BRECHT   Would you like another shot?

MARSHAL   Sure... You know, you're the first people I served a subpoena to offered me a

                    drink.

BRECHT   You're just doing your job.

MARSHAL   Exactly. But people keep movin', tryin' to avoid me... So I gotta keep chasin'

                    'em... Runnin' up and down stairs all day, knockin' on doors, gettin' blisters on

                    my goddamn feet. And when I finally do catch up to 'em, they act like

                    everything's my fault... But the people I'm chasin', they don't bother me half as

                    much as the goddamn government. This is all just a racket to get politicians

                    votes is all it is... Nothin' gets people hopped up like a threat, whether it's real or

                    not... But I got my own racket... You see, the government, they take care of all

                    my travel expenses... And I tell 'em I use my car all the time when I'm outa

                    town... But I really take the train, which costs a hell of a lot less... So I've been

                    able to pick up an extra hundred a month...tax free. And I'm savin' all that wear

                    and tear on my automobile. *(MARSHAL laughs.)* You gotta take whatever you

                    can get nowadays, whenever you can get it.

BRECHT   One more for the road.

MARSHAL   No, I can't... I gotta drive... Good luck to you in Washington, pal. *(MARSHAL*

                    EXITS.)

BERLAU   After all these years, we finally have a play going to Broadway, and now this

                    has to happen.

BRECHT   The publicity's going to help sell tickets.

BERLAU   What are you going to do about HUAC?

BRECHT	We'll rehearse. You can question me about my plays and poems, especially the more radical ones. And we'll practice until I can give the right answers.
BERLAU	How long are you going to be in Washington?
BRECHT	A couple of days...
BERLAU	I'll have our apartment all set up by the time you arrive in New York.
BRECHT	*(pause)* I bought a plane ticket to Switzerland.
BERLAU	For when?
BRECHT	The ticket's open-ended. So I'll be leaving the day after the hearings.
BERLAU	Does Laughton know?
BRECHT	No. And don't tell him. With all the spying and blacklisting going on here, it's like the beginning of the Third Reich all over again.
BERLAU	I feel as if the Third Reich's been shadowing me ever since we left Copenhagen.
BRECHT	We'll talk on the phone everyday about rehearsals. And you'll relay my directions.
BERLAU	The play might not even go to New York now.
BRECHT	Of course it will.
BERLAU	Not if you're blacklisted.
BRECHT	I'm not going to let them do that to me. And we're going to be together soon. Like we've always wanted. *(BRECHT embraces BERLAU.)*
BERLAU	Where? Up in the sky somewhere?
BRECHT	Everything will be different once we're back home.

EPILOGUE

(Washington, D.C./ New York.)

ACTOR   *(ACTOR'S voice could come from offstage.)* Washington, D.C. House Un-American Activities Committee. Brecht breaks ranks with the ten 'unfriendly witnesses' who precede him by *not* refusing to answer the central question.

BRECHT   I was not a member or am not a member of any Communist Party.

ACTOR   Brecht thus avoids prison and the blacklist. *(BERLAU finds and reads crumpled poem by Brecht.)*

BERLAU   I've longed for love engulfed by fire,

     Yet resistant to becoming ash. *(BERLAU crumples poem, lowers it to her side.)*

ACTOR   From Brecht's written statement to HUAC: *(In combat mode, ANGEL heads towards BERLAU, eventually provides here with an incendiary device, i.e., a burning cigar. ANGEL EXITS.)*

BRECHT   We are living in a dangerous world.

BERLAU   A star has fallen from Cassiopeia...

BRECHT   Our state of civilization is such that mankind already is capable of becoming enormously wealthy but, as a whole, is still poverty-ridden.

BERLAU   It is the fallen star that has struck me and ignited the fire...

BRECHT   Great wars have been suffered, greater ones are imminent. *(BRECHT continues speaking as BERLAU speaks, although he pauses for a moment prior to her final line.)*

BERLAU   Love will be *destroyed* by fire...

BRECHT   And one of these wars might well wipe out mankind...

BERLAU   When produced by a false sire.

BRECHT   The ideas about how to make use of the new capabilities have not been developed much since the days when the horse had to do what man could not do.

BERLAU   Words cannot extinguish fires. *(BERLAU ignites BRECHT'S poem.)*

BRECHT   Do you not think that, in such a predicament as we now find ourselves, every new idea should be examined carefully and freely? *(The poem continues burning.)*

BERLAU   Words cannot fulfill desire...

BRECHT   Art can make such ideas clearer...and even nobler.

FINIS

Afterword

While *Brecht in L.A.* is a work of fiction, like all imaginative works it contains points of contact with the real. One might still choose to argue that plays such as *Brecht in L.A.* blur boundaries between fiction and real life, but such arguments can cut both ways. Biographies and documentaries, for example, usually incorporate, or at least utilize, disparate sources, including letters, diaries, photographs, interviews, passages from history books. When constructing the work the biographer or maker of documentaries omits, adds, selects from, reshuffles the various sources, cutting, shaping, and weaving until some sort of coherent narrative emerges that enables the reader to feel a sense of mastery over a suddenly unified and neatly structured story. Rather than encouraging the reader to take comfort in an illusory sense of mastery, perhaps it's more truthful to show the seams of a work's construction, to create gaps, spaces which invite active participation (as Brecht often tried to do in his epic theatre), so that rather than lead the reader (like a horse to a trough) to unambiguous conclusions, the author creates a text that encourages the reader or spectator to interpret. Not a true life, necessarily, but an imagined life, truthfully composed.

I understand, however, that some readers may desire to make fanciful connections between the fictional world of the play and the real world of history until the two realms magically merge and appear to become one 'real' realm. For those whose curiosity keeps pushing them away from the aesthetic and towards the real, I briefly discuss in Appendix I some historical referents that might satisfy (or frustrate) the urge for the sort of transparent realism that *Brecht in L.A.* eschews.

Utilize the work in whatever way you choose, but please be forewarned that excessive acceptance of the fictional as the real poses serious risks, both to the individual and the world at large.

Rick Mitchell

Appendix I
Historical Footnotes, Etc.

Ruth Berlau (1906-1974) Born in Copenhagen, Berlau was an actress, writer, director, active anti-fascist, and—unlike Brecht—an avowed communist. Showing great promise for creating work that merged the imagination and political engagement, Berlau published two feminist novels, *Videre* (1935), which also supported socialist ideas, and *Every Animal Can Do It* (1940), and she founded a workers' theatre in Denmark. Berlau met Brecht in Copenhagen in 1933, and shortly thereafter she translated Brecht's *The Mother* for a Danish production. Spending more and more time with Brecht, she divorced her husband and eventually joined Brecht's refuge-seeking entourage as they traveled across several countries before boarding a ship to Los Angeles in 1941. During their complex relationship, which continued until the dramatist's death, Berlau's collaborations with Brecht included ***The Caucasian Chalk Circle*** (see below) and *The Good Person of Szechwan*, and she provided feedback on many of Brecht's other writings, including his poems. Not long after arriving in the US Berlau became frustrated with her lack of gainful employment in Los Angeles and—perhaps more importantly—with her awkward arrangement with Brecht in Santa Monica, where he kept her in a nearby apartment. Subsequently, Berlau traveled to a Washington, D.C. conference in 1942 to speak about her anti-fascist work in Denmark, and soon thereafter she accepted a job in New York City with the Office of War Information. Brecht often stayed with Berlau when he visited New York seeking productions of his plays, although Berlau was increasingly unhappy there after she became pregnant (by Brecht) and lost her job. Alone, unemployed, and possessing little money, Berlau was able to travel back to the West Coast only after actor Peter Lorre provided her with a train ticket to Los Angeles. She gave birth prematurely in 1944, lost her child a couple of days later, and eventually returned to New York, where her emotions became increasingly unstable. After a breakdown in her New York apartment in late 1945, she was admitted to a Bellevue Hospital and later transferred to a mental health facility where she underwent several weeks of electroshock therapy. At Brecht's insistence, Berlau taught herself photography and created photographic records of many of Brecht's productions, beginning with the American productions of *Galileo* in 1947. In spite of her mental illness, an increasing dependence on alcohol, and her at-times frustrating relationship with Brecht, Berlau remained strong-willed and persistent, and Brecht continued to rely on her for many things, including overseeing the Broadway production of *Galileo* in his absence. Once *Galileo* had closed in early 1948, Berlau joined Brecht in Switzerland and moved with him to Berlin, although by the 1950s Brecht—to Berlau's dismay—no longer involved her in his work and remained unwilling to get a divorce. Yet their relationship persisted. Loyal to Brecht until the end, even years after his demise, Berlau died in a fire in Berlin in 1974. For a very personal perspective on Berlau and her relationship to Brecht, see *Living for Brecht: The Memoirs of Ruth Berlau*, edited by Hans Bunge.

Bertolt Brecht (1898-1956) Born Bertold Brecht in Augsburg, Bavaria, Brecht's first play, *Baal* (written in 1918, performed in 1923), a fiercely poetic work about a dissolute young poet who continues to transgress social norms while remaining exuberant, right up until his early death, enabled Brecht to make his mark as a significant dramatist. With several more works produced and published shortly thereafter, Brecht became a major playwright and poet in

Germany by the mid-1920s and he solidified his reputation with *The Threepenny Opera* (1928), a work based on John Gay's *Beggar's Opera*, with songs adapted from the poetry of Kipling and Villon. This critical and commercial breakthrough which featured music by Kurt Weill would be the only play by Brecht to achieve great popular success. Like many artists and writers living in Germany in the early 1930s, Brecht felt increasing unease as the fascists grew in power. In order to escape the Nazis, whose tentacles continued to stretch beyond Germany, Brecht traveled with his family—his wife Helene Weigel, a great stage actress, and their two children, Stefan and Barbara—through Europe, Scandinavia, and the Soviet Union. Along the way, Brecht and company were joined by collaborator and sometime-mistress Margarete Steffin and **Ruth Berlau** (see above). Although the entire group had hoped to make it to the US, Steffin—too weak from tuberculosis to continue the trip—perished in Russia as Brecht, his family, and Berlau traveled by train towards a waiting ship that would transport them to Southern California. In Los Angeles Brecht joined a growing German émigré community which included intellectuals and artists such as Theodor Adorno, Alfred Doblin, Max Horkheimer, Fritz Lang, Peter Lorre, and Thomas and Heinrich Mann. Although Brecht was actually quite productive while in the US and famous throughout much of the world, he was unable to gain a solid footing in Hollywood, which showed little interest in the unconventional form and leftist politics of the German dramatist's writings. Nonetheless, Brecht was able to earn some money by working on Hollywood films, particularly on Fritz Lang's ***Hangmen Also Die*** (see below). Frustrated by Hollywood's commercial limitations, Brecht soon gave up hopes of working as a screenwriter and concentrated on playwriting and securing a Broadway production. His only play to be fully produced while he resided in America, *Galileo*—which featured Charles Laughton, credited with the play's translation, in the title role—made it to Broadway late in 1947 after a short, summer-time run in Los Angeles. Prior to the play's New York opening, however, Brecht was called to testify in front of House Committee on Un-American Activities (**HUAC**) (see below) in Washington, and he departed the US for good shortly after his well-received (and well-rehearsed) performance in front of the Committee. Today, Brecht's theatrical innovations—as a playwright, director, and theorist—continue to influence theatre artists throughout the world, and his work is still frequently performed. His numerous plays include *A Man's a Man* (first produced in 1926), *Rise and Fall of the City of Mahagonny* (1930), *Mother Courage and Her Children* (1941), *Life of Galileo* (1943), *The Good Person of Szechwan* (1943), and *The Caucasian Chalk Circle* (1954). Most of Brecht's writings have been translated into English and are widely available. For a thorough introduction to the dramatist's ideas about theatre, see *Brecht on Theatre* (edited by John Willet), as well as *Bertolt Brecht: Journals, 1934-1955*. There are also scores of volumes that discuss Brecht's work and his legacy, including Fredric Jameson's *Brecht and Method*, Darko Suvin's *To Brecht and Beyond*, and Peter Thomson and Glendyr Sacks' *The Cambridge Companion to Brecht*. Books that focus on applications of Brecht in the late twentieth century include Janelle Reinelt's *After Brecht: British Epic Theatre* and Elizabeth Wright's *Postmodern Brecht*. Two of the more extensive biographies written in English are James K. Lyon's *Bertolt Brecht in America* and John Fuegi's *Brecht & Company: Sex, Politics, and the Making of Modern Drama* (also published outside the US as *The Life and Lies of Bertolt Brecht*).

Elsa Lanchester (1902-1986) Lanchester, the red-headed daughter of hard-living and committed Irish socialists, was born Elizabeth Sullivan in Lewisham, England and began her professional career as a dancer and cabaret artist, performing an outrageous act in a London club run by herself and two friends. Consciously bohemian, early in her career Lanchester posed nude for photographs, studied dance with Isadora Duncan (whom she despised), and spent a bit of time as a snake dancer. Lanchester eventually appeared in numerous plays and films, at times with Charles Laughton, whom she met during a London stage production of *Mr. Prohack* (1927) in which she played the secretary to Laughton's title character. Lanchester married Laughton in 1929 and within a few years they were on their way to the US, where the couple (particularly Laughton) became popular movie actors, although they briefly returned to the English stage in the late fifties. Best known for her appearance as Mary Shelley/The Monster's Bride in *The Bride of Frankenstein* (1934), Lanchester worked in a wide variety of films—including *Lassie Come Home* (1943), *Witness for the Prosecution* (1957), and *Mary Poppins* (1964)—and she made numerous television appearances. Her eccentric and comic characters were often memorable, but Lanchester never reached the stature of Laughton, with whom she remained married until his death in 1962. For the record, it is doubtful that Lanchester ever had an affair with Brecht. In her memoir, for example, she writes that Brecht 'didn't appeal to me particularly[....] He smoked awful cigars. Whether they were the expensive or the cheap ones, I don't know. Or perhaps the passing through Brecht made the smoke come out with the sourest, bitterest smell' (p. 193).

Fritz Lang (1890-1976) Born in Vienna in 1890, Lang established himself as a major director in Berlin, most notably with the expressionist films *Metropolis* (1927) and *M* (1931). In 1934 Lang relocated to Los Angeles, where his lengthy career included films such as *Hangmen Also Die* (1943), *Ministry of Fear* (1944), and *The Big Heat* (1953). Lang and Brecht had been friends in Germany, and the director had employed Brecht's wife, Helene Weigel, in small roles in silent films in Berlin. Although he earned a significant amount of money for directing American movies, Lang felt somewhat stymied working in Hollywood. Nonetheless, he chose not to return to Germany after the war. Brecht, who worked with Lang on *Hangmen* as a writer, apparently lost some of his respect for the internationally renowned director during their collaboration because—in Brecht's mind—the immensely talented director had capitulated to the commercial pressures of Hollywood. In spite of Lang's lack of enthusiasm for much of his work in the United States, many critics consider him one of the most consistent and prodigious directors of *film noir*, an area in which he often seemed to work, even before the term *film noir* had been coined.

Charles Laughton (1899-1962) Laughton, born in Scarborough, England, established himself as an accomplished theatre actor before arriving in New York with a production of *Payment Deferred*, which had opened at the St. James' Theatre, London, in 1931. His wife, Elsa Lanchester, played his fifteen-year-old daughter, and the play had short runs on Broadway and in Chicago before becoming a Hollywood film (1932), with Laughton again playing the lead. The rotund actor quickly parlayed his stage fame into a film career that saw him playing numerous leading parts and character roles in Hollywood, although by the 1940s Laughton's star was waning as many studio executives considered him a 'ham' actor who had seen better days. Laughton, whom Brecht considered a strong, theatrical actor and ideal for the role of the

Galileo, did receive some critical acclaim for his work in Brecht's play, his first stage appearance in about ten years, although the reviews of the production (and Laughton's acting) were mixed. After *Galileo* Laughton continued working in film and television, and he took some turns on the stage later in his career, both in legitimate plays in London and as a popular dramatic reader of stories and dramatic scenes from the Bible, Shakespeare, and elsewhere. Showing that his stellar work on the English translation/adaptation of *Galileo*, which Brecht had praised, was not a fluke, Laughton radically revised James Agee's screenplay for *The Night of the Hunter* (1955) and then directed a superb production which, although a failure at the box office, remains highly regarded by film scholars. Of particular interest is the form of the movie, whose theatricality seems more in line at times with Brecht's epic theatre than with Hollywood realism. During his forty-three year marriage, Laughton—with his wife's reluctant approval—often sought sexual pleasure from men, although Laughton and Lanchester remained dedicated to each other, it seems, until the end. Biographical books about Laughton include Simon Callow's *Charles Laughton: A Difficult Actor* and Charles Higham's *Charles Laughton: An Intimate Biography*.

The Caucasian Chalk Circle. Written by Brecht with assistance from Ruth Berlau, *The Caucasian Chalk Circle* is loosely based upon an old Chinese play, *The Chalk Circle*. Although Brecht wrote the work while in exile, the play did not receive its first professional production until 1956 in Berlin. *The Caucasian Chalk Circle*, considered to be one of Brecht's greatest plays, has a happy ending, an anomaly for a Brechtian work which may be attributable to Brecht's desire to secure a Broadway production for the piece.

Galileo (not to be confused with *Galileo Galilei*, the play that characters in *Brecht in L.A.* refer to, sometimes in abbreviated fashion, and rehearse). Brecht's *The Life of Galileo* was written during 1938-1939 and first produced in Zurich in 1943. In Los Angeles Brecht worked for several years with Laughton on an English translation/adaptation, *Galileo*, which opened in 1947 in Los Angeles and then on Broadway with Laughton playing the title role. The American productions, directed by Joseph Losey (with a great deal of input from Brecht), received mixed reviews in Los Angeles and harsher reviews in New York, where the production met with less success than another play about Galileo, *The Lamp at Midnight*, by Barrie Stavis, which opened two weeks after Brecht's play. Criticism of the US productions of *Galileo* in 1947 suggests that many American critics, unable to identify some of the realistic conventions to which they had become so accustomed, were put off by the work because it didn't conform to their expectations, which were based on American realism. Brecht never saw *Galileo* on Broadway since—feeling the pressure of potential obstacles to his longed-for return to Europe—he left the US for good after his HUAC appearance. Constantly reworking his plays, even after initial productions and publication, Brecht drafted a third version of the *The Life of Galileo* in the 1950s for an acclaimed production by the renowned Berliner Ensemble (Brecht's state-supported, lavishly-funded company) which the playwright himself directed. Some critics consider *The Life of Galileo* to be Brecht's masterpiece.

Hangmen Also Die (1943). Fritz Lang, who directed this film about the Czech resistance, reportedly developed much of the story with Brecht before bringing veteran screenwriter John Wexley onboard, who worked on the script with Brecht in a Hollywood studio for ten consecutive weeks. Brecht, however, was denied screen credit, purportedly for political reasons, in spite of his protest filed with the Writers Guild, but he did receive a much-needed ten-thousand-dollar paycheck for his efforts. Ultimately, Brecht tried to distance himself from the final project, claiming that his writing had been mutilated, although a significant amount of the film seems somewhat 'Brechtian'. As James K. Lyons notes, perhaps 'more of [Brecht's] presence remains in the film than many Brecht purists would care to admit' (p. 58). For a thorough and entertaining account of Brecht's experience as a Hollywood hack under Lang, see Lyon's chapter, 'A Qualified Winner: The Film *Hangmen Also Die*' (pp. 58-71), in *Bertolt Brecht in America*.

HUAC (1945-1975). Often associated with Senator Joseph McCarthy, who passionately led the Committee's extraordinary efforts to ferret out 'subversives' in the early fifties, as well as with J. Edgar Hoover, HUAC was spearheaded at first by J. Parnell Thomas. With strong assistance from cold-war-hawk Hoover's FBI, HUAC responded to the 'red menace' by utilizing Nazi-like tactics that instilled fear in many, and rightfully so, since an appearance on the HUAC blacklist often ended one's career. HUAC's fervent, right-wing witch hunts were eventually rejected by the American public, but not until the Committee's activities had destroyed many lives. Both Brecht and Berlau, 'suspected communists', were spied on by the FBI, and Brecht was called to testify in 1947, shortly before *Galileo* opened on Broadway with Laughton in the lead. Although an often-ignored accusation by **Joseph Losey** (see below) from a 1975 interview points to Laughton as the person who denounced Brecht to the FBI, Lyons dismisses Losey's claim as 'unfounded' (p. 315). For a more extensive rebuttal of Losey's accusation see Elsa Lanchester's memoir (pp. 198-199). HUAC had lost much of its initial luster towards the end of McCarthy's reign, although the Committee remained actively engaged in its cold war mission through the late 1960s.

Mother Courage and Her Children. First produced in Zurich in 1941, *Mother Courage* takes place during the Thirty Years War and features one of Brecht's strongest dramatic characters in the title role. Believing that it in order to see the present, and ourselves, clearly, we must first develop some distance between ourselves and our objects of analyses, Brecht often sets plays in the past not so much to comment on a historical period, but to help the spectator see the present in a new, more critical light. Thus, *Mother Courage* can be read, in part, as a commentary on modern war. The famous Berliner Ensemble production of *Mother Courage and Her Children*, which featured Brecht's wife, Helene Weigel, in a widely praised performance as Mother Courage, cemented Brecht's fame as a playwright and director, particularly when the production visited Paris towards the end of Brecht's life, in 1954.

Projections, etc. All projections attributed to 'bb', as well as the lines from the play within the play, are works of the imagination by the author of *Brecht in L.A.* The play's projections related to spying, the FBI, and/or HUAC are based on material covertly collected by the US Government, which developed secret files on thousands of people residing in America during and after World War II. Much of this classified material became potentially available through an act of Congress, the Freedom of Information Act. Although the Act enables American citizens to request previously classified documents, some of the requested documents remain classified, or partially censored (or 'blacked out'), even after a request is made, so not all information covered by the Act is freely available. Nonetheless, much of the material that has been accessed under the Act, such as documentation of whom someone has called on the telephone or had sex with, makes many former American law makers and enforcers seem similar to the purported agents of totalitarian authorities whom they were supposedly striving to stifle. For an example of the sort of material that the US Government collected on the German emigre community during the mid-twentieth century, see Alexander Stephan's *Communazis: FBI Surveillance of German Emigre Writers.*

Some Brief References...

While living in New York, the English poet **W.H. Auden** collaborated with Brecht on an adaptation of *The Duchess of Malfi* and spent some time reworking a rough translation of *The Caucasian Chalk Circle.* Brecht, however, was unsatisfied with what he considered Auden's slight contribution to the latter project and Auden—unwilling to make further revisions—stopped working on the play, which remained professionally unproduced in America during Brecht's lifetime.

Edgar Bergen (a ventriloquist) and **Charlie McCarthy** (a dummy) were a popular comedy team in vaudeville, on the radio, and in the movies.

Frank Capra, who made numerous light-hearted films, such as *Platinum Blonde* (1931), *It Happened One Night* (1934), and *Mr. Smith Goes to Washington* (1939), is perhaps best known for ***It's a Wonderful Life*** (1946), a popular, sentimental film of small-town life that continues to fill American television screens during the Christmas holiday.

J. Edgar Hoover regularly utilized underhanded tactics, including spying and blackmail, as Director of the FBI, which he oversaw from 1924 until his death in 1972. Rumors persist that Hoover, publicly a homophobe, was gay and that he dressed in drag, although—remarkably— the person who oversaw the compilation of data on the sexual proclivities of countless individuals apparently managed to cover up most traces of his own sexual endeavors.

Peter Lorre, a German emigre who starred as Galy Gay in Brecht's *A Man's A Man* (1926) and Lang's *M* (1931), utilized his unique presence and considerable acting skills to create numerous memorable characters in Hollywood, although his career and life began a downward spiral in 1946 after Warner Brothers failed to renew his contract. An exceptionally literate Hollywood actor, as well as an old friend of Brecht's, Lorre developed an addiction to morphine and was often relegated to buffoonish roles towards the end of his career.

Joseph Losey first met Laughton and Lanchester on Broadway, while he was stage manager of *Payment Deferred.* Losey went on to direct several plays and films, including the 1947 stage productions of *Galileo* in America. He later directed a British film version of *Galileo* (1973) which is notable for its adaptation to the screen of non-realistic elements of Brecht's epic theatre.

Luise Rainer, an actress from Austria, began her career in stage plays directed by Max Reinhardt. Through mutual acquaintances, Rainer heard of Brecht's plight prior to his departure for America, and—although she lacked personal acquaintance with the dramatist—she signed an affidavit which permitted Brecht to enter the US in 1941. Rainer made her Hollywood debut in *Escapade* (1935) and won two consecutive Oscars, in 1936 (*The Great Ziegfield*) and 1937 (*The Good Earth*).

J. Parnell Thomas, a zealous chairman of HUAC who sought to uphold American moral standards by ridding the US of so-called subversives, oversaw Brecht's hearing in Washington and sent many witnesses to prison. Later convicted of adding phantom workers to the federal payroll and keeping their paychecks for himself, Thomas himself was sentenced to eighteen months in federal prison.

Orson Welles, best known for his film work as a director and actor, was originally going to produce and direct *Galileo* on Broadway for his Mercury Theatre, but last minute wrangling by Brecht and Laughton seemed to discourage Welles from pursuing the project further. Welles' film ***Citizen Kane*** (1941), which features numerous cinematic innovations, is widely considered to be one of the most important films of all time.

Appendix II
Performance Review of *Brecht in L.A.*

Brecht, Bobos, & L.A.
by
Ralph Leck

Rick Mitchell's *Brecht in L.A.* opened in a humble NoHo (North Hollywood) art house. The drama explores the interpersonal politics of the communist playwright and his struggles to make a living in the Babylon of commercial art, 1940s Hollywood. At one point in the drama, Fritz Lang (played by Jon Peterson) clarifies for Brecht the prerequisites for acquiring work. The US is at war in Europe and the Pacific, and consequently, commercial success is most assured via the genre of the war film. Unlike Germany's great émigré film director, however, Brecht is unwilling to accommodate to the jingoistic demands of the day. Instead of nationalistic art and affirmative culture, he proselytized on behalf of Epic Theatre. The dramatic epic he had in mind was existential and historical. Theatre should examine commercial capitalism and its cultural complexities as a prolegomena to the audience's civic transformation. This revolutionary goal set Brecht on a collision course with Hollywood and McCarthyite America. Appropriately, then, the denouement of the play is Brecht's appearance before the House Un-American Activities Committee (HUAC). Shortly thereafter, he left the United States and eventually moved to Berlin, East Germany, where he remained a theatre director until his death in 1956.

Not surprisingly, Brecht had difficulty finding work in Hollywood. By the early 1940s, the popular and critical acclaim of his *Threepenny Opera*, which opened in Berlin in 1923, must have seemed like the incarnation of a previous lifetime. Nonetheless, he pushed forward with many projects. One project, his collaboration with Charles Laughton on a stage production of *Galileo*, is the balloon frame around which the *Brecht in L.A.* is constructed. *Galileo* is about the power and inclination of irrationality (conservative Christianity) to suppress the institutionalization of reason. In this play within the play, the tension between religion and reason overlaps with another thematic dyad: the avaricious demands of commercial culture, symbolized by Hollywood, and the politics of economic equality, symbolized by Brecht. At the most abstract level, this play within the play is a vehicle for reflexivity. Mitchell implicitly poses a Brechtian question: isn't Brecht's predicament our own? Indeed, commercial banter about Hollywood's need to respond affirmatively to our current war in Afghanistan is everywhere, and Mitchell deftly explores this contemporary demand by dramatizing Brecht's resistance to what Horkheimer called 'affirmative culture'. In opposition to the hegemony of affirmative aesthetic politics, then, Mitchell offers a politics of art that aspires for poignancy without being preachy or platitudinous. The balance is perfect.

Mr. Mitchell, who also directs the play, has assembled some powerful actors. Frankly, I wasn't sure what to expect. Only days before opening night, the play was not listed on the recorded phone message of the Bitter Truth Theatre. Subsequently, it was reported that the playwright might be playing the lead role because the former lead had accepted immediate paid employment in Hollywood. True to the themes of the play, commerce invaded the realm of art. Brecht, played by Brent Blair, must have had little time to prepare for his role, but this did not negatively affect his performance. Indeed, his performance was remarkable. Brecht, the engaged artist, emerges as neither a saint nor a revolutionary buffoon. Blair's depiction, true to the script, avoids left-wing ancestor worship and right-wing demonization. Brecht emerges fully human.

Three performances—by actors who had the luxury of weeks of preparation—were riveting. First, Laughton is played brilliantly by Edmund Shaff. Hegel once remarked that Napoleon was history on horseback. Shaff's performance left me feeling as though I'd encountered an equally powerful, but different, embodiment of historical spirit, namely, the spirit of Hollywood on stage. Laughton, like Hollywood, is riven by the demands of art and mammon. We often find him coaxing Brecht to invigorate *Galileo* with commercially viable motifs, but he also is drawn to the civic insights of Brecht's dramas. Small touches, such as the way he rubbed his male lover's back with conviction and compassion, distinguished Shaff's performance. Most powerful was his use of intonation. His ascending and discriminating speech always seemed to be on the edge of theatrical decorum. It was loud, over-the-top, and thoroughly convincing.

Second, Mary Beth O'Donovan—appearing in white dime-store tennis shoes, a humble black skirt to the ankles, and a gray petite sweater—played Brecht's lover and artistic collaborator, Ruth Berlau. Berlau was a cosmopolitan European woman who had the humility and demeanor of a Mecklenberg peasant, or, at least, that's the way O'Donovan portrayed her. Berlau encapsulates the predicament of BoBo (bourgeois bohemian) culture. The cultural leaders of the European Left espoused the politics of the working class but were rarely from humble economic origins. Most, like Benjamin, Bloch, and Lukacs, possessed an upper bourgeois pedigree. In Berlau, we meet someone with reverses of cultural capital, a countercultural disposition, but limited economic means. At first sight, she appears to be exploited by Brecht. She wants a traditional life together, but Brecht still lives with his wife and children who never appear on stage. Instead of a traditional life with Brecht, she receives entreaties to translate and transcribe his work. In essence, Berlau performed the intellectual equivalent of reproductive labor for Brecht. This model of collaboration is something akin to textile enterprises that market "their" product using a company logo but without reference to the female proletariat that produced it. Although the play does not mention other examples, Brecht had a history of this type of collaboration. Elizabeth Hauptman translated John Gay's *Beggar's Opera* for Brecht but received no credit for having facilitated *Threepenny Opera*.

This leitmotif is important but dangerous. One can easily forget that Brecht rejected entirely individualist conceptions of creativity. Art is a collective and historical product that is not created *ex nihilo* by the artistic genius. There is a danger, then, that dramatic concentration on authorship, interpersonal peccadilloes, and character flaws will lead to a dismissal of Brecht's civic and artistic legacy. The writing and acting combine to avoid this pitfall. We find that Ruth is hardly an innocent victim. She willingly left a marriage in Europe to live near Brecht. If disproportionately Ruth is presented as a demur woman unjustly denied Brecht's compassion, she also emerges as a strong woman who is responsible for her liaison with Brecht and complicit in its ongoing emotional consequences.

Third, Catherine McGoohan played the role of Charles Laughton's wife, Elsa Lanchester, and her performance too was redolent with dramatic epiphanies. Her class role was that of the upper bourgeois matron. During the play, the seven principle actors were always on stage. No one contributed as much to the play while seated silently than did Ms. McGoohan. She sat on her cheap metal chair as though on an aristocratic throne but with the humility and concentration of the Buddha. Her performance, like Shaff's, always seemed on the brink of credulity. In her role, she was too smart, too composed, and too replete, and, yet, somehow she avoided caricature. Her most amazing accomplishment was her combination of action and inaction. In her latter role, she was something like a Taoist master; she miraculously projected the spiritual earnestness of Brechtian drama through the mindful act of sitting. She, more than any other actor, achieved Brecht's intention that Epic Theatre be presented as if the actors where hidden behind Kabuki masks. Elsa is the archetype of bourgeois vacuity, and McGoohan embodies her as though the role was cut to fit at a Beverly Hills boutique.

Some aspects of the play came off less well. Brecht's Cuban lawn boy, Angel, is a dramatic foil reminding the audience that Marxist intellectuals require the labor of the working class. The actor, Del Toro, played Angel without the requisite conviction of his dynamic historical role. Angel is the working-class critic who alternatively schools and scolds the left-wing artist. His insightful criticisms of Brecht's Marxism enable this exchange to be more than a cute spanking of a BoBo Marxist. Angel is a craft socialist a la William Morris. Brecht, conversely, professes an industrial vision of the socialist future that is incompatible with the preservation of craft production. Perhaps due to the impassivity of Toro's performance, this rift within socialism unfortunately did not attain the dramatic clarity that the author intended.

There is another critique of Brecht's Leninist Marxism that is inchoate in *Brecht in L.A.* Leninist Marxism assumes that women will be emancipated by their participation in public work. Consequently, unlike utopian socialists, Marxists historically have tended to exclude the reproductive labor of the domestic sphere from the theoretical and political domain of "work." And, because it was untheorized, reproductive labor was never democratized in communist countries. Women in communist countries found themselves working a second shift after returning home from their public occupations. There is a parallel in the play. True to Marxist form, the childcare and multiple domestic duties performed by Brecht's wife are displaced from this drama. Brecht's wife never appears on this dramatic stage of history.

The playwright chose to stage *Brecht in L.A.* like Louis Malle's wonderful film adaptation of *Uncle Vanya*—as a reading. In its present stripped-down form, it's an uncut gem whose brilliance will not be enhanced by additional polishing or a more fashionable setting. The fine script, superb acting, and engaging themes combine to make this a must see production.

"Brecht, Bobos, & L.A." is reprinted with permission from *Communications from the International Brecht Society*, where the review originally appeared (Vol. 31, No. 1, 2002).

Ralph Leck, a cultural/intellectual historian who lived in East Berlin prior to the fall of the Berlin Wall and in West Berlin after German unification, was a frequent visitor to Brecht's Berliner Ensemble. He recently published *Georg Simmel and Avant-Garde Sociology: The Birth of Modernity, 1880-1920*. *Brecht in L.A.* was performed as a staged reading at the Bitter Truth Playhouse, North Hollywood, California, in November 2001 as part of the Edge of the World Theater Festival, sponsored by Theater L.A.

Works Cited

Adorno, Theodor and Walter Benjamin, Ernst Bloch, Bertolt Brecht, Georg Lukacs. *Aesthetics and Politics*. London: Verso, 1980.

Benjamin, Walter. 'N [Theoretics of Knowledge, Theory of Progress]'. *The Philosophical Forum: A Quarterly*. Vol. XV, Nos. 1-2, Fall Winter, 1983-84. 1-40.

Berlau, Ruth. *Living for Brecht: The Memoirs of Ruth Berlau*. Ed. Hans Bunge. Trans. Geoffrey Skelton. New York: Fromm International Publishing, 1987.

Brecht, Bertolt. *Bertolt Brecht: Journals 1934-1955*. Trans. Hugh Rorrison. Ed. John Willet. New York: Routledge, 1993.

—. *Bertolt Brecht: Poems 1913-1956*. Ed. John Willet and Ralph Mannheim, with Erich Fried. New York: Routledge, 1987.

—. *Brecht on Theatre: The Development of an Aesthetic*. Ed. and Trans. John Willet. New York: Hill and Wang, 1964.

Callow, Simon. *Charles Laughton: A Difficult Actor*. New York: Grove, 1988.

Diamond, Elin. 'Mimesis, Mimicry, and the 'True-Real". *Acting Out: Feminist Performances*. Eds. Lynda Hart and Peggy Phelan. Ann Arbor: University of Michigan Press, 1993. 363-382.

Edson, Margaret. *Wit*. New York: Faber and Faber, 1999.

—. Fuegi, John. *Brecht & Company: Sex, Politics, and the Making of Modern Drama*. New York: Grove, 1994.

—. *Bertolt Brecht: Chaos, According to Plan*. Cambridge: Cambridge UP, 1987.

Harrop, John. *Acting*. London: Routledge, 1992.

Higham, Charles. *Charles Laughton: An Intimate Biography*. Garden City, NY: Doubleday, 1976.

Hurwicz, Angelika. 'Brecht's Work with Actors'. *Brecht as They Knew Him*. New York: International, 1974. 131-134.

Jameson, Fredric. *Brecht and Method*. New York: Verso, 1998.

Lahr, John. 'Fortress Mamet'. *The New Yorker*. Nov. 17, 1997. 70-82.

Lanchester, Elsa. *Elsa Lanchester, Herself*. New York: St. Martin's Press, 1983.

Leck, Ralph. 'Brecht, Bobos, & L.A.' *Communications from the International Brecht Society*. Vol. 31, No. 1, 2002. 28-30.

Leight, Warren. *Side Man*. New York: Grove Press, 1998.

Lyon, James K. *Bertolt Brecht in America*. Princeton: Princeton UP, 1980.

Mamet, David. *True and False: Heresy and Common Sense for the Actor*. New York: Pantheon Books, 1997.

Meyerhold, Vsevolod. 'The Naturalistic Theatre and the Theatre of Mood'. *Anton Chekhov's Plays*. Trans. and ed. Eugene Bristow. New York: Norton, 1977. 313-321.

Mitchell, Richard W. 'Creating Theatre on Society's Margins'. *Contemporary Theatre Review*. Vol. 11, Nos. 3 & 4, 2001. 93-117.

Reinelt, Janelle. *After Brecht: British Epic Theater*. Ann Arbor: University of Michigan Press, 1994.

Stephan, Alexander. Trans. Jan Van Heurck. *Communazis: FBI Surveillance of German Emigre Writers*. New Haven: Yale UP, 2000.

Suvin, Darko. *To Brecht and Beyond: Soundings in Modern Dramaturgy*. Sussex: Harvester Press, 1984.

Thomson, Peter and Glendyr Sacks. *The Cambridge Companion to Brecht*. Cambridge: Cambridge UP, 1994.

Wright, Elizabeth. *Postmodern Brecht: A Re-Presentation*. London: Routledge, 1989.

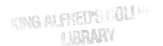

ART | FILM | TECHNOLOGY | THEATRE | CULTURE | MEDIA

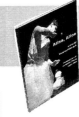

Alisa, Alice
A play by Dragica Potocnjak,
Translated by Lesley Anne Wade

This play deals symbolically with the attitude of the European Union towards refugees, and specifically with issues of prejudice between two small nations with different religions, in the immediate context of a power relationship between a Slovenian and a Bosnian woman. This translation will contribute to an understanding of the relationship between the personal and the political, and provide insights into sources of prejudice, which inhabit our own lives.

Paper, 82pp
1-84150-104-2
£14.95

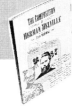

The Composition of Herman Melville
A play about writing and dramatic composition
By Rick Mitchell

The play, which contains bibliographical information relating to Herman Melville, is an explanation of the ways in which writers compose and are composed. Parallels between past and present (in racism, domestic abuse, and the plight of the visionary American artist) are clearly implied; but the play also utilizes new technologies, like video, in order to represent the kind of dialectical history and representation promoted by Benjamin.
The utilization of various performance strategies within the play generates the exposure of the complex textuality of a writer who has haunted the landscape of America from the mid-nineteenth century to the present.

Paper, 96pp
1-84150-067-4
£14.95

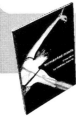

Tormented Minds
Three plays by Christine Roberts

Ceremonial Kisses • Shading the Crime • The Maternal Cloister
An anthology of three plays, each featuring a protagonist who is compelled to confront his or her particular oppressors.
Each play is very different in style. The range of techniques include the use of physical theatre, naturalistic dialogue, symbolic structures, puppets and poetry. The plays are supported by essays about the process of their development and their themes. All the plays have been produced on stage. Production photographs are included in this volume.

Paper, 137pp
1-84150-081-X
£14.95

Intellect, in association with *Studies in Theatre & Performance*, publishes new writing for the theatre (or work that is new to U.K. audiences).
The publications in this series:
- promote tolerance, cultural exchange and dialogue through theatre;
- represent work that is aesthetically and/or stylistically innovative;
- may not be considered appropriate for production by 'mainstream' venues (in that they are experimental, risky, non-commercial, thematically or politically challenging, etc.);
- include contextualizing essays or author's notes to support the performance texts.
Please submit scripts, playtexts and/or performance writings that fit the above criteria to Roberta Mock, series editor, for consideration (r.mock@plymouth.ac.uk).

intellectbooks

Publishers of original thinking. PO Box 862 Bristol, BS99 1DE, UK www.intellectbooks.com